You'll Never Believe Me, Nurse!

Kate Lesage

You'll Never Believe Me, Nurse!

© Kate Lesage 2023

Front cover designed by Abbie Smith

Shoe illustrations by Sarah Crescence

Contents

Acknowledgements   i
List of abbreviations and meanings   iii
Preface   v

PROLOGUE   1

1   LONDON
Growing up – ghosts and ghettos   7

2   BRIGHTON
Playing hide the hamster at nursing school   22

3   NEW YORK
Love rules in the Big Apple   48

4   PARIS
Real friends and faux pas   72

5   ANTWERP
Diamonds sparkle even under the greyest skies   94

6   GRENOBLE
Girls just wanna have fun (with anaesthesia)   104

7   THE CAPE
Our Love is King   117

8   FROM TWO TO THREE
A baby, stitch ups and driving fiascos   143

9   FROM THREE TO FOUR
Another baby, and a return home   166

10   BACK TO PAREE
Mismanaging the stars   181

11 HAITI
One small drop in an ocean of goodwill (and rum)   203

12 CAMBRIDGE
NHS Revisited   218

13 GENEVA
Eyes and lows   236

14 WHERE NOW?
Medication Time to Meditation Time   255

Acknowledgements

My undying love and gratitude for your help and patience, Christophe, Alex and Emilie. And also to Chris, Roger, Tom, Dad, Jo and Vik, Julia and Steven, Kev, Leigh, Estelle, Penny (and all my Old Raineian pals), Madame Donton, Anne Marie, Olive and Kevin, Helen, Julian, Joanne G, François B-L, Amel, Supermanu, Kathy, Annette, Guillaume, Colm, Rene and Maithe and all my nursing set (you know who you are!)

A special thank you to Lissa Gibbins, Justine Cunningham, Anna Maskell, Cheryl Rosebush, Liv Siegl, Damian Meaney, Stephen Clarke and all the doctors and nurses who were kind enough to share their juicy stories with me!

A big thank you to Liz Hales, Chris Hunter and Team at Amazon Publishing Pros for helping make my book a reality. Your expertise and dedication have been invaluable, and I am grateful for your contribution to this project.

Names, dates, places, stories and even personalities have been changed to protect those who, quite understandably, wish to remain anonymous. No negative judgement on any religion, sexual persuasion or race is intended.

Apart from the French, of course.

In memory of Mum.

And Alexandra, my beautiful friend.

Dedicated to nurses all over the world.

List of abbreviations and meanings

A+E – Accident and emergency department
ARS – Agence Régionale de Santé: the local French health authority
BMA – British Medical Association
CCTV – Closed circuit television
CDD – Contrat de durée determinée: fixed time work contract
CDI – Contrat de durée indeterminée: open-ended work contract
CHU – Centre Hospitalier Universitaire: French university hospital
CNED – Centre national d'enseignement à distance: national center for distance education
CO_2 – Carbon dioxide
CV – Curriculum Vitae
DNA test – A saliva test which looks at specific locations of a person's genome, therefore estimating their ancestry end ethnicity
DNR – *Do not resuscitate* in the event of cardiac arrest
ECG – Electrocardiogram
EPHAD – Etablissement d'hébergement pour personnes âgées dépendentes: medically assisted living facility for seniors
ETA – Estimated time of arrival
ER – Emergency room
FAC – Faculté: French higher education facility
FBI – US Federal Bureau of Investigation
GCS – Glasgow Coma Scale
GP – General practitioner, family doctor
HPST – A French health law called Hôpital Patient Santé Territoire
HP – Hewlett Packard (company)
HR – Human resources department
ICU – Intensive care unit
IV – Intravenous
MRI – Magnetic Resonance Imaging. A diagnostic radiology technique.
MRSA – A staphylococcus aureus bacteria resistant to common antibiotics
NGT – Nasogastric tube
NHS – The UK's National Health System
NMC – The UK's Nursing and Midwifery Council
O_2 – Oxygen

Obs – Observations carried out by medical personnel, such as pulse rate and blood pressure
PEEP – Positive end expiratory pressure; a mechanical ventilation aid
RGN – Registered general nurse UK
RN – Registered nurse US
SAMU – Service d'Aide Médicale Urgente: France's emergency ambulance service
TGV – Train de Grande Vitesse: France's high speed trains
WHO – World Health Organization

Argot
French slang, familiar language.

Bow Bells
St Mary-le-Bow is a historic church in Cheapside, London. Its bells are prominent in several famous English songs and stories. People born within earshot are considered *cockney*.

Cockney
A Londoner from the East End, traditionally proudly originating from the lower class, who has a distinct dialect of English which includes the use of word-rhyming.

Petit Bateau
Rather bourgeois French children and babies clothing range.

Stool chart
A clinical assessment tool used in Britain to help classify faeces.

Déchocage
Literally means to *un-shock*. French hospital department, where the teams manage the most severe, often life-threatening emergencies.

Preface

Whenever something incredible happens in my life, an overwhelming urge to share the experience floods over me, with the added hope of simultaneously making someone, somewhere, chuckle. Hence, I suppose, the overpowering control of today's social media. Generous nature, clown or show off? Possibly a little of each, let's be honest. For me, becoming a nurse has indeed been an incredible experience, and if you have ever wondered what it might be like working in this crazy profession, if you are already in it and seeking comparison, or are simply a curious patient, these stories are mine to share with you.

The word "nurse" originates from Latin, meaning "to nourish". Providing the energy to live nourishment comes in many forms; we need to feed our bodies, but also our minds and hearts. Nursing is fodder for the spirit – soul food. Utter heartbreak and fits of laughter are part of our daily routine. Because of this, we are in a unique position, and our unique tales deserve to be told.

This book is both a geographical and physical journey but also an intensely psychological one (often more psycho than logical). For the faint-hearted amongst you – take heed – you have been warned! But as with any voyage, there are twists, turns and unsuspected lows as well as highs. I've taken the wrong direction and found myself lost on more than one occasion. Shocking, surprising scenes and encounters have led me to the slap-on-the-forehead realisation that the human race is barmy. We are complex, captivating and endearing, yes… but also completely bonkers. Human beings are capable of the best and the worst of things. This is the very nature of freedom.

In spite of these all too human traits, my experiences have led to lifelong friendships, treasured memories and even love.

No trip ever leaves the traveller indifferent or untouched. We return home stronger, infinitely more knowledgeable, open-minded and independent. Reflecting on my own journey has been an extremely cathartic and vital personal process. *You'll Never Believe Me, Nurse!* is not *just* tales of removing foreign bodies from foreign bodies – rather the story of one person's life and how nursing influenced and changed it.

Nurses come from every background; there's no mould, no particular criteria. The common denominator *should* be kindness, but unfortunately, that's not always the case. Patients hand over their complete trust, like passengers to an airline pilot. We see them dying, naked, angry, scared. Raising people's awareness that they have the right to choose, to protection and to informed decision-making was my key motivation for this project.

Whatever brings a patient to the emergency room, general practitioner, maternity ward, retirement home, or operating theatre is always either by luck or choice (or lack thereof). Everyone, at some point in their lives, will, therefore, probably be cared for by a nurse. We are mere mortals, and there's nothing we can do about it! But what we *can* do is fight to save the NHS, to improve nurses' working conditions, including their education process. Because if we don't, we may just find ourselves in a terribly desperate and even catastrophic place in the not-too-distant future.

This precious thing called life – as nurses, we're taught to ease, normalise, improve, advance and ultimately save it. If I had to live *this* professional life all over again, would I? If I had a choice, would I take the often crap salary, red-eyed night shifts, aggressive doctors and frustrated patients? Witness the tragic death of children, deal with ulcer-inducing stress and handle disgusting bodily fluids on a daily basis? Put up with chronic understaffing, pitiful looks and terrible, never-ending back pain? I'd like to think so. But, honestly, I'm not sure.

About a year ago, I seriously considered embarking on a

complete professional change. To help me choose what on earth I could do instead and to see if I really *did* want out, I decided to look back on my career: what's to like and what's not to like – the good, the bad and the ugly parts of nursing.

Once I'd started scribbling down notes, there was no stopping me… and this book is the end result.

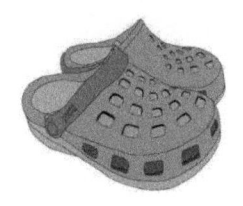

PROLOGUE

The patient was turning blue.

A nice shade, though. Almost purple, like an early autumn sky as the sun sinks below the horizon.

I stood above him, paralysed with shock. It was one of those pivotal moments in life... one you never forget, when the world stops turning for just an instant amid overwhelming feelings of hopelessness, helplessness and disbelief.

With a syringe in one hand, a metal torch in the other and an old professor's feeble erection poking into the small of my back, I swayed slightly. I forgot everything else around me and asked myself one question: *How the hell did I get here?*

How did a working-class girl from the East End of London, with absolutely no medical ambitions whatsoever, end up wandering around dazed and confused on foreign soil in that strange parallel universe known as an operating theatre? Sporting a pair of thin, blue pyjamas and sweaty, plastic clogs. Surrounded by respirators exhaling deeply into her ears like dirty phone callers. Not to mention the even stranger people.

Sniggering, whispering and even singing in a language I could hardly fathom, they moved in to form a curious circle around me, like those ominous boulders at Stonehenge. Not having the foggiest clue about what I was supposed to be doing, but with just enough sanity left to realise that there was something vaguely inappropriate going on behind me, I suddenly experienced a strong desire to run. Or start blubbing. Or both.

Which *planet* had I landed on? The answer to that one was easy.

France.

I'd already journeyed to a few foreign shores… but this was by far the most bizarre situation I had yet to find myself in.

The elderly anaesthetist was clearly making the most of his final days at the hospital before an early retirement. Forced retirement, rumour had it, after one too many cheeky remarks to female colleagues. He was the infamous Head of Department, a professor no less, and his name was Doctor Neaux (pronounced *No*), evoking visions of early James Bond villains in my panicked brain.

When I'd walked into his consultation room that morning, I'd half expected him to greet me from a swivel chair wearing shiny black gloves with a fluffy, white cat on his lap.

"B… bonjour," I had stammered. "I am Madame Lesage… *je suis la nouvelle*, the new… anaesthesia, um… student."

I was terrified. I knew that I was to be marked on my abilities; I was about to put my first-ever patient to sleep.

Cue Bond film music and flashback…

Do you expect me to talk, doctor? Ha! No, nurse, I expect you to die.

He had scrawny shoulders and a huge, gold stethoscope hanging round his hairy neck, engraved with a large N. Obviously overcompensating for something, which, no doubt should have been dealt with in earlier years. He'd looked at me over his glasses with a bemused, predatorial expression. You must understand that the French find the English accent *extremely* sexy for some unknown reason. Personally, I prefer their rolling, romantic Latin tongue to our harsh Germanic tones. Which is one of the reasons why I'd ended up in this mess in the first place.

"Aha," he'd replied, "ze new Breetish student! Keep talking ma chérie... I feel like I'm in a real-life 'ow you say... porno film?"

I bet your arse is jealous of all the crap that just came out of your mouth, I reflected silently.

Stay calm, Kate. Just imagine him on the toilet.

Dr Neaux had been charged with helping me perform my first intubation: the holy grail of anaesthesiology. This is a procedure whereby one sticks a breathing tube down into the patient's trachea (leading to the lungs) with the help of a torch-like instrument called a laryngoscope. All the time, trying to avoid the oesophagus (which leads to the stomach).

These two entrances are extremely close to each other. If any partially digested and highly acidic gastric contents somersault from the oesophagus into the trachea, they can turn lung tissue into cottage cheese. In this case, you can pretty much say *adieu!* to your patient, who would then be more likely to leave the operating room not on a medical stretcher, but feet-first in a wooden box. This is the reason why eating solids less than six hours before surgery is strictly prohibited, which includes milk, sweets, chewing gum, many fruit juices and cigarettes, by the way. The stress kicked in. I started to tremble uncontrollably.

Dr Neaux handed me a syringe of milky-white liquid and instructed me to inject it into the patient's intravenous (IV) catheter. I knew that this was propofol, the anaesthetic agent made famous by music's best-known insomniac, Michael Jackson.

"Are you going to give me a leetle cocktail, nurse?" smiled Monsieur Bichet, the unsuspecting patient, glancing at the clock on the wall, tapping his wrist and winking at me. "After all, eez time for z'apéro, non?"

It was always *apéritif* o'clock in this country.

"*Exactement!*" replied the doctor. "Zis one is called Propofol on ze Beach. Enjoy!"

With a quick push on the plunger, the patient quickly lost coherence, then consciousness, with a happy sigh followed by a heavy slump. Lucky for him, really, as at this moment, my esteemed instructor grabbed one of the scrub nurses and started to twirl her around the room, launching into a rendition of, "Eef you like pina colaaadaaa…"

Having studied the potential side effects of all the drugs I was to use, I knew that, like most anaesthetic medications, propofol could cause a serious allergic reaction.

Just as Monsieur Bichet stopped breathing and I was clumsily preparing the laryngoscope to intubate, his face blew up like a balloon at a child's birthday party. His skin was starting to resemble the French (and British) flags: pasty white, followed by all shades of blue, then dark red. I knew that the potential life-threatening diagnosis was anaphylactic shock, the redness and swelling signifying massive histamine release and blood vessel dilatation, which is the body's natural response to an allergy.

I popped an oxygen mask over his mouth and called out quickly for a vial of epinephrine: a powerful vessel constrictor which helps to get the falling pressure back up and relaxes lung spasm at the same time. My Americanism was met with total incomprehension, mixed with that traditional French mannerism: utter contempt. In France, they use their generic names for drugs. The word "adrenaline" *may* have solicited my desired reaction, but I'll never be sure.

The anaesthetist just shrugged and let out a bored "*Bof.*" He didn't seem overly bothered by the situation, having witnessed it many times before during his long career. He knew better than I did that it would most likely pass in a few seconds. To add to his indifference, the patient was not a VIP, being neither cabinet minister, lawyer nor a fellow doctor. Poor old Monsieur

Bichet was a nobody.

Being young, blond and, above all, from England, word had spread that I was easy prey. The hospital had wagered a huge risk, as well as a large sum of money on deciding to give a scholarship to someone unable to string two words of French together.

This was apparently all part of a new policy of hiring *défavorisé* or "disadvantaged" people. Along with the other immigrants, the partially sighted and wheelchairbound, I was already the target of a fair amount of curious scrutiny amongst my colleagues and classmates. I also quickly realised that everyone would attempt to speak English to me, unfortunately defeating the object of improving my abysmal grasp of this new language.

I could almost feel the burning heat on my bottom as a pair of eyes laser-beamed me from behind. Even though papery pyjamas (scrubs) are decidedly unflattering and leave much to the imagination… when one crouches over to perform the laryngoscopy it's possible, by squinting *very* hard, to decipher the outline of a pair of knickers.

Exciting stuff if you're a frustrated old quack, I suppose. It soon became apparent that upon entering an operating room, women were expected to leave their dignity in their locker, along with all other personal items.

Although Dr Neaux seemed more interested in trying to sneak a peek down my scrub top as I peered over our rapidly inflating, scarlet Monsieur Bichet, this very much felt like an emergency to *me* and I was determined not to lose my first French patient. I already had visions of myself dressed as Marie Antoinette, neck on the chopping block. Desperate to communicate with someone in the room who might actually react, wringing my hands in distress, I decided just to shout as loudly and clearly as I could manage in English.

"THE PATIENT IS RED!"

That's when Doctor Neaux came up behind me and started gyrating his groin with a big smirk.

"Me too, baybeee!"

The entire operating theatre collapsed into howling fits of laughter, some actually rolling around on the floor, totally ignoring the poor patient… who was by now turning violet.

I later found out that *raide*, pronounced "red" in French, can mean stiff or erect. So that was the end of *that* particular entente cordiale and the beginning of many years of Franglais faux-pas, cultural cock-ups and medical mishaps.

Mr Bichet, you will be pleased to hear, came out of this little episode contentedly smiling and in one piece. What's so convenient about anaesthesia is that one doesn't feel or remember a thing.

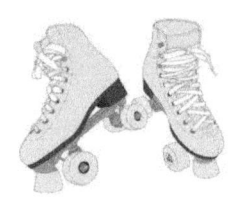

1. LONDON

Growing up – ghosts and ghettos

> Maybe it's because I'm a Londoner
> That I love London so
> Maybe it's because I'm a Londoner
> That I think of her
> Wherever I go
>
> I get a funny feeling inside of me
> Just walking up and down
> Maybe it's because I'm a Londoner
> That I love London town

Maybe it's because I'm a Londoner, Hubert Gregg (1944)

I grew up in the slum that was London's East End during the early 1970s. Born so close to the sound of Bow Bells, I still have the ringing in my ears. Looking back now, it seems aeons ago.

We lived in a dilapidated Victorian terraced house on Southborough Road in Hackney. My mum, already on her second failing marriage, was best friends with Mrs Kray, mother of the murderous Ronnie and Reggie. They had bonded over having twins. I had three smaller half-brothers, the twins being almost totally identical. The only way of telling them apart for the first five years was that one of them had a crocodile-shaped birthmark on his left arse cheek, so I only knew who was who whilst changing their terry-cloth nappies.

My dad was a psychologist of Scottish descent, whom I only saw on alternate weekends whilst growing up; Judge's orders. He had understandably moved as far away from London as possible in order to escape his strange, estranged ex-wife. Mum was an extremely difficult and scary person to live with. She spent her time between intense psychotherapy sessions, shouting at us wildly and studying for her numerous PhDs. I don't think she ever did a *real* day's work in her life, and had a hard time grasping the connotation of motherly (or indeed any other kind of) love. Following a horrifically abusive childhood, Mum was depressed, compulsive, violent, and, I suspect, borderline schizophrenic. Although she didn't have the traditional double personality; that would have been too simple. There was an entire village living inside her brain.

Unusually beautiful, extremely manipulative and having a Mensa level IQ of over 130, she was never in want of friends, admirers or husbands. I was absolutely terrified of her, and spent years and years as a child just trying to get her to like me, failing miserably.

The upside of all this was that I joined every after-school club imaginable, simply to avoid going home when the end of school bell rang. As well as library, painting and drama clubs I learned about marine biology, built bookshelves, played chess and took violin classes. I was in every single school musical production even though, as anyone will tell you, when I start to sing any nearby dogs start howling. I was on all the sports teams – again, as anyone will tell you, there's my picture in the Oxford dictionary under the definition of a couch potato.

If there was nothing going on, I'd simply hide in the toilets until the cleaners chucked me out.

There were so many wonderful indie girls' names to be had at the end of the '60s: Meadow, Saffron, Delilah… but I got lumbered with boring old Kate. They may as well have called me Kay, as no one ever pronounced the T. It could have been something worse, like Mildred, Deidre or Brenda, I suppose. One has to count one's blessings; names such as these were quite common at the time; naming your offspring appallingly wasn't questioned in those days. There was even an unfortunate girl in my primary school whose sadistic parents christened her Sausage Chips. *I kid you not.*

At least I had an interesting middle name: Rae. This originated from my paternal Highland Macrae clan ancestry. We even have our own fancy Scottish hunting tartan and ruined castle on a misty loch. *Fortitude* is the Macrae motto: to show great courage in the face of danger. A befitting phrase, growing up in Hackney.

Everyone in our neighbourhood spoke cockney. According to local folklore, this dialect of rhyming slang was initially invented to try and fool the Irish immigrants in 1900s London. The mixture of English, Scottish and cockney meant that few people understood what was being said (or rather, yelled) in our house.

A simple phrase such as, "Come inside, children! Upstairs quickly now, and wash your dirty little faces with soap," was translated as: "Git in this hoose reet noo! Up them apples and pears quick as ye can an' scrub yer darty wee boat-races wiv Bob Hope!" Bit tricky for an outsider to decipher, I grant you.

We had particular expressions for everyday words. A man was not a man. He was a bloke, guvna or me old china (plate rhyming with mate.) A woman was referred to as a bird and addressed as love, pet or darlin'. A telephone was a dog and bone. The pub (boozer) was a battle cruiser. If you were brown bread, you were dead. And "…don't forget to wash your Alan Whickers" (knickers), especially if they pen and ink (stink).

Straight up! meant you were telling the truth. Cor blimey! expressed surprise. "Don't you be tellin' me porkies" meant that you weren't supposed to lie (pork pie). To not give a monkey's signified that you didn't care. However, if you gave a monkey *to* someone, you'd handed them over 500 quid.

We could smell a non-East Ender a mile away. 'T' was something you drank large quantities of, not pronounced. Anyone who had the misfortune to pronounce theirs was a "…total toffee-nosed twat from outta taan." Try saying *that* with no Ts.

Ours was a multicultural street. My childhood was spent surrounded by, playing and going to school with, children of every shade of colour. It was so unimportant to us that we never gave it a second thought. It simply didn't matter, as, of course, it shouldn't.

Whether it was skipping in and out of a long rope in the road, jumping hopscotch onto chalked squares, splashing around at York Hall swimming baths… ringing doorbells in the council flats and running away, annoying pedestrians on our second-hand roller-skates or even occasionally getting flashed at by the perverts hiding in the bushes of Victoria "Vicky" Park, we had a right old giraffe (laugh) together.

The smells drifting out of the Bethnal Green, Whitechapel and Mile End tube stations were the same as the local public houses: stale beer, fag ends and piss. Walking past the forbidden pub doors, we would ask each other: What happened in there? Why were all of the grown-ups permanently congregated inside these mysterious havens after sunset? What dark magic converted relatively normal middle-aged folk into giggling, amorous teenagers or snarling, aggressive beasts? We tried to sneak in, of course, but inevitably got dragged straight back out by the scruff of our necks.

Climbing over bricks and barbed wire and dodging London's famously large grey rats, we would head over the waste grounds, dumps and allotments towards the canals every weekend. Mangy German Shepherd guard dogs barked and growled in our direction, foaming at the mouths and pulling on their chains. But fear wasn't enough to deter us. We'd each drag along branches, stealthily gathered from Vicky Park, in order to help us fish anything out of the smelly, dark green, algae-filled water that happened to be floating along.

We didn't have lakes, rivers or the sea. Hackney's narrow waterways were our playground. Burst footballs, handkerchiefs, bicycle tyres, shoes… everything was extracted, meticulously examined and played with before being disposed of once more into the murky depths with a loud splash.

Who did this shoe belong to? That looks like an old lady's shoe… was she dead? Gasp, shudder! Maybe she was murdered… her barefoot ghost might be right next to you. Run! Quick!

It was a smelly, noisy, frightening, exciting place where imaginations grew and story-telling developed in that magical time before television and mobile phones.

The odour of home-made chips soaked in vinegar wafted out of our kitchen windows in the evening to mingle with the smells of Jamaican coco bread, African chicken Yassa and Indian garam masala spices.

The background music to all the hustle and bustle came in the form of Boney M, Simon and Garfunkel, Aretha Franklin, the Rolling Stones, Eric Clapton, Madness, The Beatles, Gerry Rafferty, The Jam and Bob Marley, to name but a few. A musical mixture as colourful as the people listening to it. I shall never understand people who are intolerant of skins other than those of their own shade. In my opinion, considering the British Empire's colonial past, it's more than a teeny bit hypocritical to complain about sharing our country with different cultures. Growing up in an inner city was tough without a doubt, but it was there I learned that a world void of social melting pots would be unimaginative, soulless and sterile. The music would be pretty boring, too.

My best friend at primary school was called Rhianna. She was stone deaf, and she taught me sign language, focusing, obviously, on the worst swear words. Very useful indeed for slanging matches with the hard of hearing, even today. Her stepfather was a dark, handsome New Zealander called Blair. He had wild, curly black hair, a permanent smile plastered on his bearded face, alongside infinite patience.

I spent my summer holidays with them on the island of Malta, driving down in their rickety Volkswagen camper van through France to catch the thirty-hour ferry ride from Salerno, Italy. These vacations were my annual escape from London and my happiest childhood memories.

Blair was buddies with Dominic Mintoff, the then-socialist Maltese president. We would sit on the flat, pink-stoned presidential residence rooftop under the stars, playing with adorable Pluto-type guard dogs, relishing blood-orange *gelato* and juicy prickly pears stolen from the palace gardens. Listening to the adults discussing Marxist ideology on the terrace below, the crickets chirped into the small hours amid the perfume of lemongrass, jasmine and dope. It was a world away from home.

Our days there were spent endlessly jumping off the rocks at St Paul's Bay into the warm, turquoise Mediterranean. We swam for hours amongst the yellow and blue-painted fishing boats, diving down, holding our noses, to catch starfish and sea urchins, which would then spend the day ineffectively attempting to crawl up and escape out of our cheap, plastic buckets.

Doe-eyed and open-mouthed, we'd stare longingly at the shirtless boys on their Vespa scooters, lads who didn't look twice back at us pasty English lassies. There was no way we could compete with the beautiful, dark-haired, suntanned island girls. Being "friends" of Mintoff, however, we didn't have to pay for our bus fares, cold drinks or ice creams. The *xarabanks* took us all over the island. These brightly coloured, uniquely customised buses had music constantly blaring out at full volume – Diana Ross was a favourite of that era – as they charged down the dusty roads; hundreds of fake-bejewelled

Catholic crosses dangled from every bus roof and swung in our faces. As we held on for our lives onto the seat in front around every cliffhanging turn (seatbelts didn't exist in those days), everyone sang merrily along to *My Old Piano*, *Ain't No Mountain High Enough*, and *I'm Coming Out*.

These happy times came to an end in 1979.

Blair… this wonderful, gentle stepdad, partner, teacher and friend, was bludgeoned to death by a police officer in an anti-racism protest. Just because of his political convictions and foreign looks. Fourteen people witnessed the murder, yet no one has ever been brought to justice. I remember being very young, attending the long funeral march and walking next to my weeping friend as we sang Lennon's *Imagine,* overwhelmed by the sad incomprehension of it all.

Many years later, I read a story about a black man in America who was shot dead running away from the police. He was just jogging. *Jogging*! Sometimes I feel so sad that nothing has changed. No lesson has been learned from Blair's unnecessary, untimely, avoidable death. There are good cops and bad cops, of course – good nurses and bad, likewise – but the baddies should be weeded out and punished, not allowed to hide behind the mostly virtuous ones.

I came to believe that life is pretty much determined by three things: where you are born, what your parents do for a living and, most importantly, what colour your skin is.

My parents spent what little money they had on repairing our house, which was falling to bits and infested with mice. Our garden resembled a dump, in the middle of which permanently stood a large, yellow skip. I shared a small room with my brothers, but this was nothing compared to the Indian family next door: there must have been sixteen or seventeen of them; we lost count.

Unless you include the runny mince at school, meat was eaten once a week in our house (either tinned spam or roast chicken, the best parts being viciously fought over) for tea on Saturday. Our staple diet was chips, chips and… more chips. A rusty, pale- blue Ford Cortina with no wheel caps was parked outside on the rare occasions that it hadn't been stolen and taken off on a joy ride. It coughed black smoke and made so much noise clanging down the road that I always lay flat on the back seat, face down, in case someone from school spotted me.

We had no new clothes, no real birthday parties and rare presents. Our Christmas stockings were a pair of Mum's old tights cut up, holding a few walnuts, a tangerine and a Terry's chocolate orange if we were lucky. When the ice cream van came chiming noisily along our street, my brothers and I ran after it as if we were following the Pied Piper, drooling over the idea of the ultimate culinary delicacy: a vanilla Mr Whippy with a "99" chocolate flake pushed halfway in and covered in *monkey blood* (strawberry sauce). Never having the money to actually buy one, we could only jealously watch the other kids tucking in, sweet cream dripping down their cornets and chins. Our only real treat was the occasional packet of salt and vinegar crisps to share between siblings as we waited patiently for our parents in various pub gardens at weekend lunchtimes.

Looking back, however, despite the odd hunger pain, permanent embarrassment at the state of my shoes and clothes, and the fact that every single thing we owned came from a second-hand auction sale, I never *really* wanted for anything material.

Just as pub culture was the norm in those days, so were drugs, the swinging sixties being just over our shoulders. The men were bearded, the women braless. My parents and their friends dressed in flowery skirts, large, pointed collars and flared jeans, a joint permanently being passed around the bean- bags.

Crime was also rife in 1970's gangland London. My family stopped getting mugged in the street once the muggers realised we didn't have anything worth pinching. But burglars were everywhere; it was a popular career choice at the time. It was 1975, and mum had just bought our first telly; a black and white 10×10-inch screen with a wire coat hanger for an antenna. This was by far the most exciting thing *ever* to have happened in our lives. My brothers and I sat hypnotised for hours in front of *Blue Peter*, *Little House on the Prairie* and *The Magic Roundabout*.

The Magic Roundabout! What was all that about? A bunch of animals permanently stoned out of their heads, hanging around a fairground all day. They were not really the best role models, but we loved them. It's like my other somewhat questionable favourite afternoon programme: *Captain Pugwash*.

"Captain! Where's Master Bates?"
"Tossing in his bunk again, probably."

But the halcyon days of children's cartoons weren't to last long in our house. One afternoon, I was sitting in our living room watching *Scooby Doo* when two men with stockings over their heads appeared, unplugged the TV and calmly proceeded to carry it away. I was still in a state of shock when they came back moments later, rolled the carpet up under my feet and took that, too.

We were too poor to go to the hairdressers, so Mum would put a bowl upside down on our heads and simply cut around it, often chopping off a bit of ear in the process. Thank goodness Joanna Lumley came along as Purdy in *The New Avengers* and made the style trendy.

We had strict instructions not to use more than one square of crackly, thin, hard toilet roll on each visit to the loo. And, yes, Mum counted! Woe betide any of us using more, even if we had a dose of the squits. If we were caught, we would then be presented with our usual choice of punishment: stick, belt or slipper. I cheated by stealing nice, soft paper from the school lavatory dispensers and kept it rolled up, hidden in my pencil case for emergencies.

Mum used to make sure that my brothers and I were in bed by 6.30 p.m. every night so that she could skip off down to the pub. When word got around, gangs of kids from my year used to come and throw stones at our house after she'd gone until I came to the bedroom window in my flowery nightie, whereby they would gleefully wolf whistle at me.

"Not coming out tonight, Kate? You look lovely!" Guffaws of mocking laughter. "There's a disco down the estate… *come on!*" "I can't. Now, bugger off!" I would draw the curtains together, red-faced with humiliation. I'd have loved to go to discos with the other kids… but if I dared to disobey Mum, there'd be hell to pay. I was angry and ashamed but never felt real hatred towards any of them. Despite everything, we were somehow all in it together. I wasn't the only one with money and parent issues. There was a strong sense of underlying East End community spirit and a strangely powerful (completely non-academic) allegiance to our school. The badges on our blazer pockets made us part of a pack, ready to beat any different badge-wearer to a pulp. It was a jungle out there; we taunted each other daily, snarling those well-known words through thin lips, fists clenched:

"Come an' 'ave a go if ya fink yer 'ard enough!"

School was a red-bricked, austere building surrounded by a high wall and barbed wire to avoid escape. I succeeded quite well academically during my first few years, even though I hated it with a vengeance. It was almost an hour's walk every morning and afternoon down the Mile End Road to and from neighbouring Stepney. We walked because my brothers and I kept the intended five-pence bus fare in order to buy tooth-rotting sweets – one pence pear drops, black jacks and flying saucers being our favourites. As our bus drove past, the cool kids in the rear seats made obscene gestures, both to pedestrians and to the drivers of the cars behind. Our area was so rough that being up on the top deck was almost like going out on a safari. Observing people fight like animals was as normal as watching a window cleaner or lollypop lady.

Long before the existence of ISIS and al-Qaeda, it was the era of IRA attacks. Bombings in London were a regular occurrence during the '70s and '80s. Their favourite target seemed to be our public transport system. Whenever I took the bus or a tube, I was never certain to get off it alive. It made for strange times, days when we were grateful for the slightest things, mainly just getting through them with all four limbs still intact. On the occasions when we were too tired, or it was raining too hard, we did catch the bus but jumped off in-between stops at thirty miles an hour without paying, the conductor angrily shaking his fist and hurling obscenities at us. Red double-deckers in those days had an open platform at the rear where you hopped on and off. This was later abandoned for obvious safety reasons.

None of the classes at school interested me other than art and English. I was too shy to put my hand up for fear of getting it wrong. *Yes, miss, please miss, no miss…* that wasn't in my nature. My hormone-saturated, daydreaming brain was focused on one thing and one thing only: boys.

My first kiss was aged eleven with Andy: a short, ginger-haired boy in my class who nobody else fancied. It happened behind the canteen in the bike shed at the end of the playground: the designated place for smoking and snogging. We walked around hand in hand for a while after that. This was called "going out" and was considered a very serious thing. He took me to see my first films at the Hackney Empire cinema, where he groped hopefully around at my flat chest on torn, red velvet chairs in the darkness. We watched classic Hollywood gold such as *Grease*, *Strange Encounters of the Third Kind* and *Rocky*. I whimpered into the safety of his arms during the terrifying bits in *Jaws* and the scary *Swarm* with its evil killer bees.

Gangly, clumsy and unprotected by absent parents, I was systematically and mercilessly bullied, along with so many others. Physical violence and intimidation were part of kids' lives way before the onslaught of Twitter and Facebook. Schoolchildren in those days were arranged into groups according to strict hierarchical rules. At the top of the pecking order were the gang leaders: the ones with tough parents, such as policemen, local criminals and pub landlords. Children having parents who were considered useful: sweetshop owners or a man-with-a-van, were also quite high up on the scale.

All these kids were to be respected, and they carefully picked out members of their *own* subgroup: the strongest, best-looking, most daring and insolent being first choices. Even head teachers didn't have the guts to mess with top gang members on the odd occasion that they actually showed up for class for fear of getting their tyres (or even necks) slashed. Children such as myself were at the bottom of the pile. Always the last to be called to join a team in sports, no pocket money to share/steal and bits of curtain sewn into our second-hand clothes at the knees and elbows as unsightly makeshift patches. At least wearing a uniform meant that ostentatious financial differences were minimised. But then all you had to do was look downwards where the shoes would give it away.

School, like home, could often feel threatening and unsafe. Heads were flushed down toilets daily, and compass stabbings were commonplace. Even a few of the teachers hit kids for absolutely no reason in those days. Whenever I was caught staring out of the window daydreaming instead of doing boring algebra exercises, I'd get a ruler abruptly slapped down over my knuckles. Or dragged by my ear into the corner, hunched shoulders turned away from my fellow students in shame for the rest of the lesson. In the end, I got used to being beaten up at school and ridiculed at home, and, far worse, sometimes simply ignored at both.

My dad had given me a second-hand new-fangled music

machine. It was all the rage at the time: a tape player/recorder called a Sony Walkman. From that moment on, it was stuck almost permanently to my ears, and the crazy, nasty outside world simply faded away. When the bigger kids tried to pinch it off me, I fought like a cat. No way was I losing this precious treasure to some thug.

John, a friend at school, told me about a group he liked. They were called Japan. The first time I heard *The Other Side of Life* bordered on a religious experience for me. Something suddenly made life beautiful and worthwhile. The haunting, deep voice that belongs to David Sylvian was, and still is to me, the sound of an angel singing. In any case, it saved my tortured soul on more than one occasion. My favourite song of his was the eerie, atmospheric *Ghosts* which somehow spoke straight to my heart. It sounds silly, perhaps, but I didn't feel alone any more. Someone else understood the painful suffering I felt and had put it into words.

Instead of taking the easy road by siding with the bullies or totally drowning in self-pity, I learned to run fast, hide well and make people laugh. I also lost myself in hundreds of Rudyard Kipling, Roald Dahl and Enid Blyton books. Blyton's boarding school tales sounded like heaven to me. Imagine not having to go home! I wrote my own stories, too, mostly fantasies to do with finding out I was adopted. The cribs at the maternity had been mixed up, and my *real* mother was scouring the earth to find me. In my mind, she had open arms, a kind smile and was holding out a double vanilla Mr Whippy dripping in monkey blood. Most importantly, I made friends with nice people. People I still keep in touch with today.

Someone I know who grew up in my neighbourhood got bullied atrociously, much more severely than most. In spite of that, he has done extremely well in life. He's happy, he has a lovely family and has travelled around the world. He became a successful lawyer and now runs his own company. He went back to Hackney years after we left school and got in contact with the kids (now middle-aged) who had beaten him up so badly that he had been hospitalised for months. He arranged to meet them one by one. He received hugs, tears, and sincere, desperate apologies from all of the lads. He realised they were not kids from joyful, safe places but had grown up themselves in violent homes, were craving attention and hiding in groups behind bullies' masks, scared of becoming the victim themselves.

Without wishing to condone violence, in hindsight, I believe that growing up in that harsh, cruel environment prepared me (and others like me) for the big, bad world… teaching us to be assertive, appreciative, respectful of authority and open-minded. Streetwise… yet tolerant and understanding at the same time. Later on in life, I was totally at ease living in seemingly dangerous places, such as Harlem, and not easily shocked by life, which can certainly be a bonus in nursing. Occasionally, when things got really, really bad and I couldn't see a way out, I *would* find myself half-tempted to chuck myself off the top of the neighbouring block of flats or swallow a handful of Mum's pills. But then I would find a reason to carry on, listen to Mr Sylvian's melodies and have faith in a better future.

With the onset of Mum's second, particularly nasty divorce, however, rebellion reared its ugly head. Her shouting, threatening and throwing eventually evolved into kicking, pushing and slapping. My stepdad moved out, and Mum's drinking got worse. She even fermented her own beer in the bathtub; the house reeked. I had to wash myself and my little brothers shivering at the toilet sink with a shared, tattered flannel.

I was fifteen and started skiving off school, wandering along the King's Road plastered in my mother's makeup. I hooked up with a bunch of hippies who offered me weird roll-up cigarettes. We stole beers from corner shops and sat drinking together, dragging on disgusting home-made soggy joints, listening to

Prince on a ghetto blaster amongst the curious squirrels in Regent's Park. I barely turned up for school and did no homework at all, spending more time waiting outside the headmaster's door and in detention than in class.

Running away for good, in the end, was the only solution when the verbal violence towards me became increasingly physical, too. I was big enough to defend and look after myself now. I spent my nights crashed out on friends' floors, on my dad's sofa bed or, even occasionally, a park bench. I constantly worried about my brothers and my pet hamster, Mitzi. But by some miracle, I passed my art and art history A-levels. I was eighteen. Skint, alone and confused… and at a total loss as to what to do with my life.

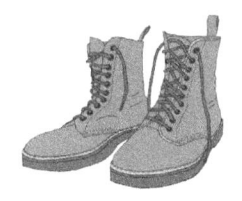

2. BRIGHTON

Playing hide the hamster at
nursing school

You may wonder, quite rightly, why on earth *anyone* would want to be a nurse.

Over the years, I've heard many answers to that question. The most common one being, "It sounded like a good idea at the time."

"My mum was a nurse," was familiar. Or "I want to help people."

A few found the idea of rarely being faced with unemployment somewhat reassuring.

Several of the prettier girls were on a mission: *Gonna marry a doctor*. Give any spotty geek a white coat, hang a stethoscope around his neck, and he immediately metamorphoses into quite a catch: your quintessential lifesaving heartthrob who probably even drives a Range Rover.

Gay men were in abundance, looking for a compassionate and tolerant profession. Straight men were onto a good thing, almost completely surrounded by young, single women. For them, it was like being a kid in a sweet shop with unlimited pocket money to spend.

I fell into nursing in a different way.

I'd been messing around at a second-rate university in London; that sometimes pseudo-intellectual, slightly pretentious place that the majority of eighteen-year-olds think they should end up at but where only a minority really belong. I certainly didn't.

I quickly realised that few of my fellow students emerged before lunchtime and that everybody did the strict minimum as far as lectures were concerned. It was easy to get a mate to sign the attendance form for you. Then, all that was left to do was snuggle back down under the duvet for an afternoon nap before hitting the campus bars for cheap beer in the evenings, all the while maintaining a haughty superiority to non-university goers.

History of Art was my subject of choice, as I had judged it the easiest through which to bullshit my way into getting a degree. Despite the delights of the Italian Renaissance and Dutch Impressionists, I spent most classes half-asleep due to a mixture of cheap beer-induced hangovers and intense boredom.

I was working in a pub after lectures to make ends meet. My dad came in one evening and mentioned to me, as I was monotonously filling his pint glass, that nursing students got paid during their studies: two hundred pounds per month plus free accommodation. The time it took me to calculate how many nights out a week I could get for fifty quid was about the time it took me to make my decision. Dad thought this was a great idea and said he'd help me out financially whilst waiting for my first paycheck. He even bought me a bicycle, my first proper means of transport.

I applied to and was accepted at Brighton Nursing School. The interviewer, a bald man in his fifties who'd come all the way to London to meet potential candidates, was head of the nurse education department. He acknowledged that my CV wasn't particularly nurse-worthy, but we chatted, hit it off and made each other laugh. Looking back, I believe he could sense I was lost. But also kind, energetic and not too daft. He thought about it, weighed up the risks and decided to give me a chance. Years later, when I started to interview people myself as a clinical manager, I tried to remember that not everybody applying for the job necessarily ticks all the boxes.

I'd chosen Brighton as it was a cool, colourful seaside town not too far from home, renowned for its great club and music scene. And how can you not love a place that has a beach with two piers, one of which was sold for a quid, a shoe shop called *Our Soles* and a gay beauty parlour named *For Skin*? These were the days of the Beastie Boys, the Eurythmics and the Housemartins, who hung around town. Later, I would be amongst the first to experience the genius of the mighty Fatboy Slim, who in those days was called Quentin, going out with a fellow nurse and a lowly pub DJ down in the Brighton Lanes. We used to stalk the poor fellow, gazing up adoringly at his mixing deck from filthy floors, pints in hands.

I thus left tedious academia behind and headed south for the real world, chugging out of Victoria Station with all my worldly belongings in a Sainsbury's brown paper bag and a small suitcase. Leaving the grimy capital, the train entered endless ear-popping tunnels and passed dusty ivy and graffiti-covered brick walls and innumerable identical suburban backyards before heading out across the fields of Sussex. Seeing open sky and trees for the first time in ages, I felt uplifted and positive. The feeling only increased the closer we got to our destination. As we approached Brighton, a beautiful 19th-century viaduct appeared out of nowhere. Houses dotted the hillsides like freckles on undulating faces, and the promise of the seaside was in the air, brought by the sudden salty smell and hundreds of swooping, screeching gulls. Once on the bus heading up Elm Grove hill towards the hospital, I caught a glimpse of the sparkling sea. The driver told me that on a clear day, you could see all the way to France, the place that would years later, become my second home.

One of the nursing tutors, Edith, was there to meet me at the hospital entrance. She gave me a tour of the wards and services, briefly explained the curriculum and the training schedules, and handed me my first month's planning, or *off duty*, as it was called by the staff.

The block of flats at Brighton nurses' accommodation was full, so I was instructed by Edith to take my belongings to a house just outside the hospital grounds named The Cottage. The Cottage was old and dingy with a green-tinged, red-tiled roof. It was in the middle of a small park, and I saw that the lights were on downstairs as I wheeled my suitcase over the scrunching pebbles. I opened the door and took off my shoes, noticing the colourful carpet was damp underneath my feet.

I passed through a kitchen decorated in ghastly brown flowers and beige 1950s tiling. There was an empty *Blue Nun* wine bottle holding a half-melted candle on the table; the ultimate in student decoration. The musky walls in the hallway were crumbling, and the glass panes in the windows were paper-thin, but it was a palace compared to the halls of residence at uni or a bench in Vicky Park.

The only heating came from a small gas fire in the living room, embedded into what used to be a beautiful, white Victorian fireplace, huddled around which I found my new housemates, Joanne (Jo), Julia and Robert, all first-year students, like me. We immediately hit it off. They were welcoming, warm, kind – and made me laugh till my cheeks burned and tears streamed down my face.

Julia was a Londoner too, a very pretty, bubbly brunette. At our nursing school integration the following day, we all had to introduce ourselves. The serious one (imagine Bree Van De Kamp from Desperate Housewives) put her hand up and said snootily:

"My name's Daphne. I gave up a place at Oxford so that I could devote my life to looking after *normal* people less fortunate than myself."

Mimicking sticking two fingers down her throat, Julia

whispered in an American accent: "Miss Goody Two-Shoes makes me want to barf!" My favourite ever quote from my favourite ever movie: *Grease*. I have loved her unconditionally my whole life since that moment.

Jo was stunning, always in a good mood and had a soft West Country accent, originating from near Bath. She was ubertrendy, could party anyone under the table and be as fit as a fiddle in the morning. But she was always calm, gentle and motherly. Nursing suited her perfectly.

She teamed up Doc Marten boots and miniskirts with an old-school blazer. Her ash-blond hair was in a short bob, a style that set the trend for the whole town. Jo was the one who made sure that Julia and I stayed out of mischief. Not always an easy task! Especially during our European inter-railing student adventures (but that's a whole other story). She later became godmother to my lucky children.

Rob was a tall, witty Mancunian. He'd come south, looking for "a change of air," the real reason being that he was running away from a jealous fiancée, a number of other ladies and a handful of angry husbands. But why this choice of profession? Watching porn movies with titles like *Naughty Night Nurse Threesomes,* along with too many Benny Hill and Carry-On films, had a lot to do with it. He could do a great Frankie Howard: "I say, steady *on*, Matron!" His favourite chat-up line was: "If you come down to the morgue with me darlin'… I'll show you a stiff." You'd be surprised how often it worked…

He was a down-to-earth guy, though, devoid of arrogance despite coming from an extremely wealthy family. He drove a dark blue, open-top Jaguar which he'd been given by his parents as a going-away present. It was the flashiest car I'd ever seen. What with his smooth looks and a cool set of wheels, The Cottage turned into a female Piccadilly Circus before long. We made a pact between us never to complicate things, opting to remain just good friends, despite an obvious mutual attraction. This was a wise decision; his friendship turned out to be amongst the most valuable of my life.

Although I was tremendously excited about my new choice of study, the reality of nursing was not at all an easy option. *Au contraire*. Three and a half years of intense living and learning is a long time. Close, supportive relationships were vital. Apart from the exams, assessments and assignments, we discovered the hell that was night duty. When it was my turn, my teeth were stained yellow by the gallons of black coffee that I consumed to try and keep awake. On days when one of the others had worked all night, we crept around on eggshells so they could sleep.

If it wasn't a night shift, it was an early morning shift. Some days we wouldn't even get a break. We became witnesses to complete strangers' lives from before birth to after death. Our aim was to observe, absorb and repeat the tasks necessary for caring for sick fellow human beings. Achieving this would take us on a journey that stopped at every emotional station. Our travelling companions were young and old alike, physically or mentally ill, sometimes simply destined to survive or perish.

I was to experience the ecstasy of helping to save lives, bringing new ones into the world and alleviating suffering. But, in parallel, I was also to endure the agony of seeing people losing their battles, suffering horribly, or leaving life behind too soon. Illness and disease are frequently random and unfair and sometimes, unfortunately, unbeatable adversaries.

I would slowly but surely discover a new personal satisfaction in using my energy to try to impact other peoples' lives in a positive way. It's a cliché, but just holding someone's hand, giving a smile, a hug or a kind word, can make so much difference to a potentially negative, scary or painful experience.

Suddenly, I felt useful.

I quickly learnt that every patient must be treated with equal respect and care. This sounds obvious, but faced with a convicted sex offender handcuffed to a stretcher who's broken his hand in a fight, an extreme right-wing racist politician who needs a colonoscopy or a woman with chest pain wearing a necklace made entirely from the lion's teeth that she slaughtered on a hunting trip to Africa… staying neutral, stoic and polite isn't always easy. One question in our final examination was: "Is nursing an art or a science?" "I'm not interested in intellectualising compassion," I answered, "that's what nursing's all about." They passed me, anyway. Looking back, I believe it's actually a little of both; we have to be scientists *and* artists.

I fell rapidly head over heels in love with the weird environment of bedpans, dressings and specimen pots. Maybe this profession filled in my emotional gaps, making up for a childhood pretty much devoid of affection. Being part of a close-knit team was like a family of sorts, and every sweet, elderly patient was the grandparent I'd never known. I was genuinely happy and perfectly content for the first time ever. But being poor was hard. I had little financial help from my parents and was far from alone in that situation. The fifty pounds salary that had initially seemed such a huge sum soon got swallowed up in essentials: makeup, clothes and entrance fees to clubs.

Every month I'd buy a huge paper sack of potatoes and a few cans of beans. What with the candle, supper resembled a peasant's banquet from the Middle Ages. To avoid starving, I just ate what the patients didn't finish and benefited from subsidised lunches in the hospital cafeteria. For luxury items such as tampons, shampoo and Cadbury's Dairy Milk, shoplifting was the answer. Cigarettes were bummed off the rich kids like Rob and Daphne. As for alcohol? Easy. We waited for the slow dances to come on in the clubs, then simply went round the tables emptying everyone's glasses whilst they were snogging, totally unaware. Also, turning on a bit of the old Kate charm often got me a beer or two. The suckers.

Never a Saturday night went by without going *out* out. Brighton was (and still is) an incredible place to party. The pubs and clubs were always full of laughter and great music. Venues such as The Gloucester, The Escape and Dr Brighton's were a welcome change to dodgy places with dodgy names like Cinderella Rockefeller's and Dirty Dick's in London. More hours were spent getting ready – giggling, gossiping and glugging from a bottle of cider with The Cottage gang – than actually being out on the town. Once inside the clubs, you would inevitably find many of Brighton's nurses in the men's toilets bitching about everyone, cackling with laughter and sniffing amyl nitrate (poppers) with the gays; this vasodilating substance was sold openly and cheaply in sex shops during the '80s. It made you laugh till you peed your pants, but the headaches afterwards were horrendous. We were young, stupid and totally oblivious to the danger.

Sunday mornings were dedicated to finding the missing of the group, usually having fallen asleep under a hedge or on a roundabout somewhere. Once we'd found them, the hangover cures were rolled out. We'd tuck into an Egg McMuffin and fries in Churchill Square before heading off to the seafront to play *chicken*: leaping just in time, millimetres away from the huge, cold waves, as they crashed onto the sea wall. Or shopping-trolley racing along the pier. On reflection, it's a miracle nobody drowned or got arrested.

If we were ever stuck for a night out, the solution was simple. Someone in the nursing flats would burn their toast intentionally, setting off the fire alarm. The brigade would soon arrive, sirens blaring, blue lights flashing, crashing through the front entrance, hoses in hands. The swinging wooden doors would then shut, the only way of opening them again being by digital code. They were thereby locked in and forced to spend the evening with us. The firemen didn't seem to mind too much after a few drinks, and generally, no regrets were had.

We went from A to B in Julia's old, brown Mini Cooper. It needed jump-starting every time. The handbrake didn't work, either; she had to put two bricks behind the back wheels to stop it from rolling down to the seafront. The seats were full of empty cans, biscuit crumbs, cigarette butts and old crisp packets. I remember once it got stolen; the police found it abandoned on Beachy Head, and the thieves had actually hoovered it clean. We loved that car. It meant freedom. It carried us to work and to play: past the white, shingle beaches, across the downs, to the best Hawaiian burger place in Hove, to the cinema at the Marina, to our favourite fish and chip spot, The Mini Whale in Lewes. To and from parties in Worthing and Eastbourne... we even made it as far as London once. Sometimes we just drove around the narrow roads of Brighton's town centre wearing fake Ray-Bans with the windows rolled down, pretending to be "...*on patrol*..." It was a sad day when that little car died. Dabbing the tears in her eyes with a hanky after an emotional speech, Julia solemnly abandoned the Mini right at the end of the Royal Sussex Hospital underground car park, where it still is today, as far as I know.

Rob and I walked onto the main medical ward for our first placement together, shaking in our pristine starched white uniforms. Scary Sister Horton gave me instructions to clean the sluice, and "Nurse Robert" was told to assist a rather elderly and extremely constipated gentleman. I got down to scrubbing as Rob wheeled Mr Davis towards the ward toilets. For the next forty-five minutes, we could hear high-pitched wailing sounds mixed with loud grunting and pushing. At last, the wheelchair reappeared, holding a smiling Mr Davis.

"Great news, everyone," announced Rob, "it's a six-pound baby girl!" Our cheeky charmer from Manchester never got into trouble with the sisters or matrons at the hospital during our many years there. Mainly because he slept with most of them.

We quickly learnt the routine and fell in line. From the

beginning, I found the work both interesting and rewarding. In those days, we had time to really care for our patients, and we got to know them well over each two-month placement period, often becoming very fond of them.

Rob and I felt terribly sorry for one of our diabetic patients who had been told he was to have both legs amputated. Poorly controlled diabetes can harden peripheral blood vessels, leading to limb loss, coronary disease and impaired eyesight. He quite understandably fell into a deep depression, no longer eating or even accepting visitors. The only thing that made his eyes light up was the sight of Rob's Jag in the nurses' car park, visible from the ward window.

"Fancy a spin, do you mate?" asked Rob one day. The patient looked up, a wide smile slowly forming across his face.

"Do you think we could? Man, I'd love to feel the wind in my hair before the chop."

"Don't you worry," Rob said, winking in my direction. "We'll sort it."

The plan was that I would be a decoy for Sister and the other staff nurses. I'd pretend to faint in the middle of taking a blood sample while Tiny Tim (our colleague on the adjacent ward) pulled the curtains around the patient's bed and removed his drip and monitoring machines for a very long, pretend "bed bath". Rob and I were to wheel the patient to the linen lift at the other end of the ward and then down to the car park.

We managed to pull it off.

Our patient had an amazing time. Rob even let him drive with the top down, Pink Floyd blaring from the car speakers while racing along the sunny seafront. He started eating again after that and recovered well from surgery. It was obvious to us, even in those early days, that one's state of mind affects one's physical health. In retrospect, we had taken a massive risk. If we'd been caught, they'd have thrown us, immediately and unceremoniously, out of the school. But we never regretted it.

Nursing is who you are… not just what you do.

We were to be confronted with all *kinds* of tricky, sticky situations. During our emergency room placement, we were witness to many unusual problems, often involving bottoms. The patient almost always began their explanation with, "You'll never believe me, nurse… *but…*"

Training in Brighton, Europe's gay capital in the 1980s, there remained very little that I couldn't believe. The Pet Shop Boys, legend has it, for example, were named after a favourite pastime in the Brighton area involving rodents and marigold gloves. One wonders at what point the gerbil, rat or hamster realises that its new master is not actually going to put it in a lovely cage with a shiny new wheel. Things are about to get a bit claustrophobic, dark… and rather smelly.

Whenever I listen to *West End Girls*, I think of little Mitzi, my childhood companion, and my eyes well up. Apart from the obvious cruelty, one has to wonder if this eternal quest for alternative sexual gratification couldn't be otherwise obtained. Maybe sex shops should start a line in cuddly animal toys? After all, more Rampant Rabbit vibrators have been sold in Britain than there are actual bunnies in the countryside. PS. Be warned. Despite every vow of the Hippocratic Oath, those x-rays will end up on YouTube one day…

Romping around with rodents *can* lead to collateral damage. A famous tale was leaked from an American hospital around this time after two men had been admitted to A&E: one for the removal of a rectal foreign object, the other for third-degree facial burns. Apparently, man number two was checking on Hammy the hamster's activities inside man number one, using a wide tube with the aid of a cigarette lighter to illuminate the scene… when, unfortunately, man number one farted. I don't think the poor hamster came out in one piece, either.

The entire Christmas Day of my second year of nursing school was spent dealing with a young lady who required help removing a trout from her privates. The trout came out quite quickly once it had suffocated and stopped flapping around. It was the scales that proved difficult and time-consuming. I had never realised before just how many scales a trout *has*. Her boyfriend had apparently presented her with this romantic Christmas gift as proof of his affection. A word of advice, girls: if he offers you a raw fish instead of a piece of jewellery, turn and run out the door – faster than you can say sushi.

Mind you; jewellery can be equally as hazardous. A very well-endowed male patient came in one day with a tight metal band around his member. Don't ask me why. Apparently, this is known as a cock ring. The guy was in agony – in his excited state, the band was cutting off blood circulation. It looked very much like an overripe aubergine. This predicament took all the skills of Dr Williams (our perspiring house officer) to get the metal contraption free using a miniature saw and clamp without turning the patient into a eunuch. To his everlasting dismay, Dr Williams became known as "Lord of the Rings."

A typical conversation in A&E – the best place to practice interviewing techniques, a poker face being essential – often went something along the lines of:

"Just so we can understand how this all happened, sir, how did this raw potato end up inside your rectum? Once again, of course, this conversation is strictly protected by medical secrecy." The secrecy probably lasted less time than it took our on-call surgeon to remove the damn thing, which had already started to germinate.

"First of all, nurse… you're *never* going to believe me, but…"
"Don't worry, sir; we are all professionals here and have

actually already extracted... uhm... odd objects from... odd places before."

"Well, OK then, this is how my current situation played out: I had arranged for a few friends to come over for dinner, so I decided to cook my speciality, *gratin dauphinois*."

"A delicious dish. Please, do carry on."

"It was quite unlucky because my kitchen sink was completely blocked, so I decided to use my bathtub to wash the potatoes instead."

"Very unlucky indeed. What happened?"

"Because I hadn't had a wash yet today, I thought I'd peel them while taking a bath. Kill two birds with one stone."

"Pretty smart! And then?"

"I got in naked, obviously. But, rather annoyingly... because of the mixture of starch and soap, I suppose, the tub got very slippery. I fell backwards onto my bottom right on top of this big King Edward. And *that* is how it got inside me. Unbelievable, right?"

"Yes, unbelievable indeed. Not your lucky day for sure. So, no *gratin dauphinois* this evening then?"

"No, unfortunately, I have had to cancel my dinner party and spend the evening here in this blasted hospital instead. I'm starving, by the way; do you think you could bring me a sandwich?"

By law, any property must be returned to its rightful owner before discharge. He limped away a little later on, clutching his potato in a hospital pharmacy paper bag.

The following night, I cooked cauliflower with my baked beans. I felt like a change for some strange reason.

People put all kinds of nutrients into their back passages. It's almost as if upon opening the kitchen cupboard or fridge,

34

lonesome folk become overwhelmed with desire. It takes a love of food to the next level. A drag queen came in once, whose opening words were, "Ooooh nurse... I've been a *very* naughty girl with a cucumber."

One day, a guy arrived with a bottle of tomato ketchup up his backside.

"I was doing the shopping, nurse... you'll never believe me," he started.

I sat down all ears, grabbing my chart and pen, ready for yet another fascinating story.

"But when I got back from Sainsbury's with all my bags, I realised I'd locked myself out!"

"Uh-huh."

"So, I decided to shimmy up the drainpipe at the side of the house in order to open an upstairs window and let myself in."

This was going to be good.

"Unfortunately, on the second floor, I lost my foothold and fell off, landing straight onto my shopping bags and... a Heinz ketchup bottle."

As we prepared for the extraction procedure, I noticed that he was wearing jeans (not a kilt) and also that, miraculously, he hadn't suffered *any* other injuries at all after falling from a two-storey building. Oh, and on examining the aforementioned tomato ketchup bottle, we noticed that the top had been stuck on firmly with Sellotape. Bottle tops are forever getting lost...

On another memorable occasion, the on-call team were awoken at 2 a.m. in order to remove a large, muddy carrot from a 100-year-old widowed, retired vegetable farmer. "Experimenting," he announced. "To celebrate a century of life! I didn't want to die without trying it *once* you understand, nurse." He was in a bit of a state; bless him. Trying to tease it out at home with two spoons hadn't done the trick; it just made everything all the messier.

Another patient tried to convince us that he had "fallen"

onto a courgette which had been sticking up out of the ground whilst pruning his rose bushes. My medical colleague, tired and fed up, rolled her eyes at him and explained that she was a keen gardener herself, grew courgettes and knew very well that they grow horizontally, not vertically. I tried not to smile. *You've been busted there, mate.* Without batting an eyelid, he defiantly folded his arms, lifted his chin towards the heavens and stuck firmly to his story. The large, black dildo that popped out *after* we'd removed the courgette was a little trickier for him to explain.

My favourite was the guy who arrived with a tangerine thrust so far up inside that it required surgery to remove. He looked at me straight in the eye and simply said, "I don't have any explanation. Just get the effing thing out. Pretty please, nurse, with sugar on top."

After a while, all this "boys and their toys" stuff became quite mundane. We students also began to recognise the amateurs from the professionals when it came to hiding objects in questionable places. The favoured item for first-timers was a bottle. They tended to go for Coca-Cola in the 237ml glass form. The beginner's mistake was to put the narrow end up first. This may have *seemed* logical… until you want to pull it out. Good luck with that. Hence the relatively large numbers of young men we saw in the emergency surgical ward with temporary colostomy bags.

They then slowly graduated to the one-litre bottles. Or other, more varied gadgets. A household favourite was the common hoover. Probably because of its versatility: it can be used as per the bottles *or* as a suction device. I realise that *Do not put your penis into the vacuum pipe and turn it on* may not necessarily be written on the instruction leaflet, but please don't do it anyway, guys. There's rarely a happy ending.

I remember a rather pompous, well-to-do looking gentleman telling us he'd been "fiddling around" with his wife's expensive Dior deodorant (meaning he'd wedged it up his back entrance).

"It's not my fault if she doesn't perform her bedroom duties enough to satisfy me. That bloody woman spends far too much of my money on all those lotions and potions anyway…" The poor proctologist was about to go home, it was nearly 10 p.m. He wearily put on another pair of sterile latex gloves. "At least this time, it might smell nicer than usual," he reflected out loud.

"You might feel a bit of a prick," I said, inserting the patient's intravenous needle into his arm. Then, under my breath, "But I'm sure that's nothing new, is it?"

The creativity was endlessly impressive. Another patient came in with a large pestle (of mortar and pestle, the stone device for crushing herbs) well and truly lodged up where the sun never shines. After the brief operation to remove it, he said he needed it back to crunch up his wife's medication. So could we please wipe it down and give it to him discreetly upon leaving the hospital? Our kind medical secretary, Susan, took pity on him and agreed to meet on the stairwell at 6.30 p.m., just as she was finishing her shift. When it got past 7 p.m., and there was no sign of the patient, Susan telephoned him, fed up with lurking around and getting strange looks on the stairs. Her kids and husband were waiting for her at home.

"Oh, hello," he answered. "I forgot to tell you, but actually, I've changed my mind. I'm worried about infection, you see. Hospitals are so dirty. You can keep it."

"You know what?" She replied, "I'll send it to you via the post and that way, you can take it… and shove it right back up your arse."

Nurse training in those days consisted of a mixture of ward assignments and classroom instruction. Each speciality lasted about two months: medicine, surgery, gynaecology, oncology, paediatrics, accident and emergency, community, psychiatry, geriatrics, theatre and recovery. Intensive care placements were kept for post-registration. The minimum work experience of a year was deemed a requirement, which I believe was a wise decision. Newly qualified nurses shouldn't be put in situations too difficult and stressful to handle – any more than they already were.

We were taught using Maslow's hierarchy of needs as our base, the pinnacle of the pyramid is self-actualisation (personal accomplishment being more important even than food, warmth or safety). Our tutors also used Virginia Henderson's model based on her need theory, focusing on patients' interdependence and inclusion in their own care. The idea behind this was to keep hospitalisation time to a minimum.

We learnt to follow procedures and make protocols using a team approach. We also learnt how to assess a patient from head to toe, formulate a care plan based on their needs, implement the actions and constantly re-evaluate the outcomes. Focus was on psychological, social and spiritual needs as well as biological ones. The essential qualities required of us were: respect, kindness, punctuality and empathy. We were taught to question ourselves, take the initiative and be honest if we made mistakes. We had to be able to prioritise, anticipate problems and gather information, using verbal as well as nonverbal communication. Our new knowledge of anatomy, physiology and pharmacology simply complimented all of this. Just looking at a person or touching their skin can tell you *so* much. We were often told to go and find a patient willing to chat, to sit at the end of their bed for ten minutes, and then come back to the classroom. The student with the maximum amount of information won.

We studied the poem, which, legend has it, was written by an old Scottish lady in a care home on her last days before dying and then discovered by one of the nurses who was going through her meagre possessions. Whoever wrote the poem, it helps to reflect on their words if ever we become frustrated with someone elderly, who is not moving fast enough or becoming forgetful. Remember that everyone was young, once…

*What do you see, nurses, what do you see,
what are you thinking when you're looking at me?
A crabby old woman, not very wise,
uncertain of habit, with faraway eyes.*

*Who dribbles her food and makes no reply
when you say in a loud voice, "I do wish you'd try!"
Who seems not to notice the things that you do,
and forever is losing a stocking or shoe.*

*Who, resisting or not, lets you do as you will
with bathing and feeding, the long day to fill.
Is that what you're thinking? Is that what you see?
Then open your eyes, nurse; you're not looking at me.*

*I'll tell you who I am as I sit here so still,
as I do at your bidding, as I eat at your will.
I'm a small child of ten with a father and mother,
brothers and sisters, who love one another.*

*A young girl of sixteen, with wings on her feet,
dreaming that soon now a lover she'll meet.
A bride soon at twenty – my heart gives a leap,
remembering the vows that I promised to keep.*

*At twenty-five now, I have young of my own
who need me to guide and a secure happy home.
A woman of thirty, my young now grown fast,
bound to each other with ties that should last.*

*At forty my young sons have grown and are gone,
but my man's beside me to see I don't mourn.
At fifty once more babies play round my knee,
again we know children, my loved one and me.*

*Dark days are upon me, my husband is dead;
I look at the future, I shudder with dread.
For my young are all rearing young of their own,*

and I think of the years and the love that I've known.

I'm now an old woman and nature is cruel;
'tis jest to make old age look like a fool.
The body, it crumbles, grace and vigour depart,
there is now a stone where I once had a heart.

But inside this old carcass a young girl still dwells,
and now and again my battered heart swells.
I remember the joys, I remember the pain,
and I'm loving and living life over again.

I think of the years – all too few, gone too fast
and accept the stark fact that nothing can last.
So, open your eyes, nurses, open and see,
not a crabby old woman; look closer – see ME!

(Anon)

Our training didn't only take place on the wards or in the classroom. One afternoon, we were let loose in Brighton town, twenty-five crazy blindfolded nursing students, in order to "experience the difficulties of getting around and about for the visually impaired." It was terrifying – for the general public as much as for ourselves. On another day, our tutors organised a similar experience for us, this time all in wheelchairs; less dangerous, they said. And it was. Apart from when we removed Rob's brakes and sent him off with a shove down North Street, screaming towards the sea.

Understanding the teamwork necessary to run a hospital was an important part of our education. Each tiny cog in the machine is essential and merits equal respect. Nurses, midwives and doctors immediately spring to mind, but there are hundreds of different professionals, each as vital as the next, all working to make the hospital run smoothly day and night: pharmacists, paramedics, cooks, porters, auxiliaries, technicians, IT staff, cleaners, human resources personnel, radiographers, clerics and laboratory workers, to name but a few.

During my training, I discovered more about the history of

our healthcare system, which we all take for granted. The NHS is considered by some as Britain's greatest achievement. It is a system publicly funded by taxes (National Insurance), created after World War 2 in order to offer excellent healthcare to all, regardless of wealth. Primary healthcare providers make referrals to more specialised sectors. Today, 10% of the UK GDP is spent on the NHS. It is offered to anyone who has been in the country longer than six months. Every citizen has access to a General Practitioner (GP), and some services are private businesses contracted out to the public. Commissioning boards decide which services a population needs.

The smaller, private hospital sector is extremely expensive, and prices can be subject to the patient's past medical history. Surgical waiting lists in public hospitals are long, and you are not guaranteed to see your GP on the same day as the demand. At the time of writing, a staff nurse's salary averages £33,000 per year. Specialist nurses, of which there are many kinds, as well as GP practice nurses, can earn a lot more.

As we became second, then third-year students, we gained confidence and autonomy. We also made life hell for the new intakes, as those before us had done. Sniggering, we'd send the poor souls running to the hospital pharmacy holding an empty syringe for 10ml of "emergency air, please", or to theatres to ask for "a long weight."

We told one poor lad in his first year to accompany a body to the morgue in the basement. I had lain down on the stretcher and covered myself with a sheet. Once he was next to me in the lift, I sat bolt upright, making a loud "Whooo!" He didn't actually die of fright but came pretty damn close.

Nursing often requires creativity and imagination. During my psychiatric placement alongside another student, Caroline (placements were always in pairs), we encountered the lovely Mrs O'Donnelly, an elderly Irish lady who was mad as a March hare, twinned with being in the throes of Alzheimer's. She was convinced that she was the baby Jesus and that we were all conspiring to *get* her.

"It's a beautiful morning, Mrs O'Donnelly; how are you today?" we'd ask, gently turning her to face the mirror, a very un-Jesus- like reflection peering back.

"Yer forking *id-yets* the lot o' yer!" she'd yell at us. "I'm not Mrs O'Donnelly, I'm the Messiah." It was like something out of a bad Monty Python sketch. She was also refusing to do anything, notably, take a bath or shower. Stubborn as a mule, for days, she resisted all coercion, persuasion, and enticement. We had to move to Plan B. Her room was indeed starting to smell like a manger, with more than a whiff of donkey urine and goat droppings.

Mrs O'Donnelly was a devout believer, and her conversation focused entirely on biblical references, so we decided to go with this theme. We dressed Caroline in a hospital sheet, looped over her head, toga style. Turning the lights down low, she approached the patient.

"Hello, Jesus! I… am your mother, Mary."

Mrs O'Donnelly looked up. We had her attention now. "I *command* you to go forth and cleanse yourself!"

Usain Bolt couldn't have made it to the bathroom any faster. Mrs O'Donnelly came out smelling of roses, and our work was done for the day.

Choosing this profession is not for the faint-hearted. By this time, I'd witnessed everything from dingleberry bushes to colostomy crabs. The only thing capable of shocking me by now, was a defibrillator.

Every so often, we'd get a new set of medical intakes known as House Officers. This always caused much curiosity and excitement, in (the rare) case that there might be a few good-looking ones for a change. These poor guys and gals were thrown in at the deep end without armbands. Completely lost, they counted on us to show them the ropes.

"Excuse me, nurse, can you show me how to put in an NG tube? Does this ECG look dodgy to you? Urine's not supposed to be *green*, is it?"

We never questioned their credentials, trusting the hospital administration implicitly. Until, that is, the day we got a call from the local psychiatric unit. A patient had escaped and was on the loose; we should all be on the lookout. Pictures were posted around the hospital of a young man with long brown hair, wild eyes and a Dali-style moustache. He was spotted in the X-ray department. Turns out he'd snuck in with the other new doctors, pinched a white coat and had been hanging around the wards telling surprised patients about his alien abduction rectal examination experiences.

After that, we had to wear ID badges, photos of us all dangling round our necks. This particular brilliant idea was ditched after a badge fell into an open abdomen during a wound inspection.

Somebody's mugshot staring up from a mass of small intestine wasn't a pretty sight.

As all good things do, our three-and-a-half wonderful years came to an end. We had made it, although we did lose a few fellow students along the way. And not just on roundabouts.

Tiny Tim (actually over seven feet tall) was willing and able to obtain anything illegal for the right price. He was sweet and charming. Our very own Del boy.

"If you ever need drugs, a cheap car or another A-level, Kate, give me a call."

He eventually got caught and hauled away in handcuffs.

Daphne, predictably, got engaged to one of the senior

surgical registrars with a double-barrelled surname and decided to ditch nursing to be a housewife/charming hostess/boring old fart. Stacey and Jennifer realised quite early on that it wasn't the profession for them and switched over to midwifery. Hannah, a quiet, unassuming girl who'd always kept herself to herself, got busted one night at the nurses' home by Special Branch police. They found her room packed full of the stolen items that had been reported by patients and hospital staff over the previous few years. It looked like a regional branch of Oxfam in there. So, another one bit the dust.

Of the original twenty-five, the remaining twenty of us took and passed our final exams and were rewarded with what we'd so long dreamt of: replacing our plain, white paper hats for ones with a big blue stripe; we're talking *major* status symbol. Nobody in the hospital messes with someone wearing one of those.

Along with an upside-down "fob" watch pinned to our blouses, we were now also authorised to wear a silver buckle in the centre of our belts. O joy! Some saw this as a sort of buckle-measuring contest and went to extremely expensive lengths to get the most elaborately decorated, antique ones. I just had the simple clip that the NHS gave out for free. There was no more timid scurrying around now; we sashayed down the wards like Beyoncé on a catwalk.

I remember the first time I picked up the work phone with a hesitant, "Hello? *Staff nurse* speaking!" I felt overwhelmingly happy, proud… and not just a little relieved. Our tutor, Julie, used to call me her little goldfish. She said I had a memory span of about 2.6 seconds. "Lord knows how you passed," she said. But she was glad I had.

My first job after qualifying was on the urology unit at Brighton General, aka the Willy Ward. Even today, it remains one of my favourite professional memories. The patients were almost all adorable gentlemen of a certain age, bringing with them (along with their juicy prostates) lots of juicy stories to tell about the war. These old guys were real heroes; I took my new stripy hat off to them.

Happily, most urologic conditions are somewhat annoying but benign. They usually just need a bit of surgical trimming; it's like grating a rather large parmesan cheese. The symptoms of an overgrown prostate are urgency, nocturia and frequency, meaning patients need to go to the loo very often to pee, which is especially annoying at night. When all of this becomes unbearable, the patient who has been saying for months, "I'll *never* do that. My bottom is an exit, not an entrance!" is admitted to our ward. The diagnosis is via a PR (Per Rectum) examination, otherwise known as a "finger up the bum". Not everyone necessarily enjoys that, even in Brighton.

When they come back from theatre, the patient has a three-way urinary catheter with massive quantities of continuous saline irrigation hanging above them in order to prevent blood clots from forming in the bladder. The catheter can come out once the urine turns from dark red to pink to clear, generally after about three days. The problem was the clots. The little buggers. Whatever we did, however fast the irrigation flowed, we couldn't always stop them. When a clot forms, it blocks the catheter tube, so the bladder fills up to the size of a basketball in a matter of seconds, causing the poor patient to howl in agony. This requires immediate aspiration. I spent the first six months post-training running from one gentleman to the next, aspirating clots like crazy with a syringe the size of a baby's arm, completing the equivalent of about ten marathons. Beating those slimy, red blobs was incredibly satisfying.

I loved the work, I loved my patients, and I loved my colleagues. And so, although an opportunity arose that I just couldn't turn down, it was a really tough decision to leave. Once you handed in your notice in those days, your delightfully thoughtful co-workers pondered long and hard over ways to organise your departure in the most inventive manner possible. A hospital is like one big family. And, as in all families, there are always one or two evil sadists.

A few days before I was due to finish, despite being on full alert due to nagging suspicions, I was ambushed. Four or five of my aforementioned "lovely" colleagues jumped on me in the sluice room, covering my head with a pillowcase. I was dragged to the ground, kicking and screaming, and stripped down to my T-shirt and knickers. Someone put their hand over my mouth to shut me up as I felt something cold and wet being wrapped around me from my feet upwards. I was getting plastered, but not in the usual way. After a few minutes, the white bandages were as hard as a stone. I had been mummified into a sitting position with my legs together, the only holes being for my nostrils.

I felt myself being dragged into a wheelchair, taken out of the hospital and bundled into the back of a parked van. My stifled yells were ignored; the music was turned up loud enough to drown them out. We drove for a good hour before stopping and starting with increasing frequency. I remember needing to pee so badly.

From all the noise, I guessed we were in a fairly large town. Eventually, the van came to a halt, and I was hauled out. Someone pushed me along for a few minutes, and then I heard the sound of footsteps running away.

So, there I was… blindfolded, bandaged from head to foot and in a wheelchair. I could make out people moving around me and heard laughter and the clicking of cameras. I realised where I was when I heard the unmistakable chimes of Big Ben. The bastards had abandoned me right in front of Parliament. Several hours later, a sympathetic policewoman painstakingly cut the plaster off, showed me where the station showers were and even lent me a pair of inmate pyjamas. I sheepishly called dad to come and pick me up.

Needless to say, my last few days in Brighton were spent sulking profusely. I found out eventually that Robert had been behind the whole idea. Years later, organising his stag night, I had my revenge. He ended up on a ferry in Calais on the morning of his wedding, with the mother of all hangovers... and no eyebrows.

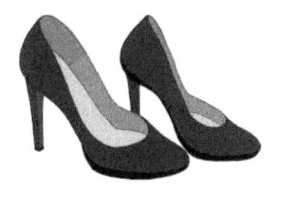

3. NEW YORK

Love rules in the Big Apple

Around six months after I'd started working in the urology department, a colleague had begged a favour of me, and I unwittingly accompanied her to a job interview at a very posh London hotel. They were recruiting nurses for the United States. My fellow nurse was hesitant about accepting the position that they were offering her in New York (having met The One down the pub the night before), which didn't seem to greatly please nor impress the interviewer.

Exasperated, he turned and instead offered the job to the person sitting next to her: me! Which is how I inadvertently found myself hired as an emergency room RN (US-registered nurse) at a busy, prestigious Manhattan hospital at the ripe old age of twenty-two, with hardly any former experience at all.

A little worrying if you think about it. Which, of course, I didn't.

I'd always longed to see America, and here was my chance. I'd spent my childhood dreaming of being Laura Ingalls from *Little House on the Prairie*. And my adulthood? Lucy Ewing from *Dallas*. To me, America was soda pop, high-school proms, drive-in movies and cheerleaders. A world away from drab old Hackney. Everybody seemed happy and beautiful in that country. I was sure that both my hair and breasts would automatically triple in size if I could just make it across the

Atlantic Ocean.

The monthly pay almost added an extra zero to my meagre NHS paycheck – it was just too good an opportunity to turn down. An RN earns an average of $80,000 a year but can increase this substantially by working in places like Los Angeles or New York, doing night duty or by agency travel nursing. When you compare this to a resident's (US house officer) salary, which is around $66.000 a year, Americans obviously consider their nurses to be vital professionals worthy of a very respectable wage. Unlike in the UK, where we content ourselves with an abysmal income after more than three years of tough training, difficult conditions and unbelievable responsibility. England was dreary and grey, full of dreary, grey men. What the hell, I thought. *Sex in the City* with George Clooney sounded good to me. Take me there!

An agency arranged everything: exams, visas, accommodation and transport. I was told to meet another nurse, also hired for the ER, in the departures lounge at Heathrow Airport; we were to travel together. At first, I mistook her for Sesame Street's Big Bird. Sitting amid a pile of yellow feathers, wearing thigh-high black leather boots and holding a tall, colourful cocktail sat Edwina McDougal from Edinburgh (aka Edinburgh Eddy). Imagine a mixture of Rita Hayworth and Cameron Diaz.

Ironically, I'd never met anyone less Eddy and more Patsy (fans of Ab Fab will understand). She was larger than life and hungry for adventure. Unlike me, she definitely wasn't looking to fall in love.

"I'm nae exactly a man-eater," she explained in between sips of Cosmopolitan. "I just chew 'em up and spit 'em oot."

By the time we landed at JFK, we had shared the stories of our lives amid squeals, giggles and more than one miniature G and T. The raucous laughing, singing and dancing in the aisle while crossing the Atlantic didn't appear to amuse everyone on that first flight, unfortunately. But we were already firm friends.

We were also blacklisted from Virgin Airlines for twelve months.

A beautiful, voluptuous redhead, Eddy had an insatiable appetite for life. Hard-partying was her religion. She was a devout believer, and I was easily converted. Our favourite deity being Bacchus, of course, the god of wine. Eddy exuded wild energy and cool style wherever she went. She had dated more than a few famous pop stars (well, snogged them on their tour buses) which proved handy in getting into New York concerts and club VIP lounges.

The music in the '80s and '90s was incomparable. It was the era of Queen, Simple Minds, Prince, Fleetwood Mac, Talk Talk, Tina Turner, Genesis, Michael Jackson, Madonna, Oasis, Whitney Houston, U2 and David Bowie… it just doesn't get *any* better. Looking back, I feel so incredibly lucky to have been young at that time. And Eddy and I shared a major passion for music, especially acid jazz. With my new bestie, we went backstage at Jamiroquai, Big Country, Simply Red and Del Amitri. We yelled and screamed so loudly that we were sometimes dragged up on stage with the band; one of my best music memories was rocking and clapping right alongside the B52s at Jones Beach on Long Island. I'd never met anyone else who loved The Brand New Heavies more than I did. Eddy also introduced me to US3, Guru, MC Solaar, Dawn Penn and Mary J Blige.

"I may be a wee bit pale and freckly on the outside," she purred. "But honey, inside… I'm *pure* black."

Eddy confided that she'd gotten into big-time trouble at Edinburgh's Royal Infirmary. Particularly hungover one morning and feeling too nauseous to stand up and take the patients' observations (pulse, blood pressure, temperature etc.), she'd done it sitting at the nurses' desk with a slightly green complexion. Writing down Mr Smith's imaginary blood pressure as 140/75 and Mrs Jones' temperature as 36.5°, Eddy was later called into matron's office. She was asked to explain why a patient who had died at midnight suddenly had a normal pulse at nine o'clock in the morning.

"Is that why you had to leave Scotland and come to America?" I asked her.

"Och no, hen," she replied, "*that's* 'cos I was caught smooching a polytraumatised patient in full traction on the orthopaedic unit."

Once in New York, we graduated from Topshop totty to Chanel chic. Babycham to Bollinger. Toast and marmite to truffles. Poppers to pure cocaine. For anyone desirous of this revolting white powder, it was literally flying around Manhattan's avenues in the early '90s like snow on a blustery mountaintop.

British nursing staff were in high demand overseas in those days and, as I said, extremely well paid. After years of reading INSUFFICIENT FUNDS at the cashpoint, I now had thousands of dollars in my account that I couldn't spend fast enough.

I was to work in what was affectionately known as the ER. "Zoo" was a more realistic and appropriate term. After a few months there, I understood why we were all foreigners: no self-respecting American nurse would even consider it. In this ER, about 20% of us were Brits and Aussies. The other 80% were mostly gay Filipinos: divas mincing around the ward with an attitude by day, flamboyant drag queens mincing around on a stage by night.

George Clooney lookalikes were nowhere to be seen either – that fantasy quickly evaporated. Most of the medical personnel were strict Jews, totally uninterested in non-Jewish girls such as myself. I wasn't particularly bothered. One whiff of a ringlet reminded me of Nellie Olsen, Laura Ingalls' nasty, blond arch-enemy in *Little House on the Prairie*.

The hospital gave us accommodation in the halls of residence on 106th Street and Madison. Built-in the '70s, they were small rooms covered in mock-brick wallpaper, housing little more than a short, rather uncomfortable wooden bed. There was a basic kitchen and bathroom to share between five of us. The other three girls were Catholic, vegetarian, non-smoking teetotallers: this was a seriously no-fun zone. The evenings' activities consisted of Scrabble, Pictionary or Monopoly. We called them *bored* games, much to the (un) amusement of our new flatmates. Eddy and I quickly started searching Midtown East and found our own tiny, one-bedroom place to rent in Murray Hill. There wasn't enough room in there to swing a cat. I slept on a mattress in the living/kitchen area, but it had a great view, being twenty-seven floors up, and there was even a rooftop pool.

When we weren't working, I ambled around with Eddy and the gang of British ex-pats, along with a few cool Australian nurses and doctors with whom we'd become pals. Together, we explored East Village blues joints, Harlem's African restaurants, Upper West Side Irish bars and Soho nightclubs. The rest of us girls contented ourselves with taking a back seat to all the male attention Eddy attracted. Favouring tailored trouser suits with nothing but a lacy bra underneath, twinned with kitten heels, she had a style all of her own. Strangers on the street would regularly get down on one knee and ask for her hand in marriage.

She also somehow knew where all the hidden, happening places in the city were as if she had some secret in-built city guide. I didn't ask questions, just followed along. We plodded past graffitied walls, deserted school playgrounds, parking lots and Korean delis with their shiny, waxed fruit on display. Up and down gusty avenues, filthy subway stairs, ear-popping elevators and brownstone steps. All amid wolf whistles followed by "Yo, hot babes!" or, "Y'all want coke or smoke?"

Walking down 10th Street one warm evening, for example, she stopped and knocked on a grey metal door which had no writing or doorbell on it. It looked as if the building was derelict, abandoned.

"What the heck are you doing, Eddy?" I asked nervously. "There's no one here!"

The door slowly opened, and a huge bouncer looked down at us, drawling, "Sorry. Private invitation only this evening, ladies."

Without skipping a beat, putting on her best sad dog eyes and poor lil'ol'me expression, Eddy replied wistfully, "Och, but we're *nurses…?*"

The guy sighed, then opened the door wider to let us in, and my jaw dropped. The place was a huge, magnificent baroque-style loft with a twenty-foot ceiling decorated in luxurious red velvet curtains, eighteenth-century Spanish paintings by Goya, and crystal chandeliers. Thrones were dotted around instead of chairs.

"I hope this isn't some dodgy S and M place," I muttered, images of The Gimp from the recently released *Pulp Fiction* still fresh in my mind.

As we made our way over to the bar amongst the beautiful and wealthy, I noticed a tiny person curled up on one of the thrones, surrounded by an adoring crowd of onlookers, kneeling at her feet.

"Oh my God, Eddy," I gasped. "Look… it's Her Majesty, Madonna!"

We didn't muster enough courage to go over and say hello to our idol. We simply spent the night worshipping her from afar. And going to the loo every five minutes in the hope of bumping into her, which we never did. She was probably using the men's.

I "bumped" into Madonna on only one other occasion during my stay in New York. I was walking down 59th Street with a friend, and we came across a gaggle of people who seemed to be just milling about, waiting for something. Noticing the red carpet leading from an adjacent cinema, we decide to hang around behind the ropes too. Just in case.

It happened to be the premiere of *Sleepless in Seattle*, a romantic comedy starring Tom Hanks and Meg Ryan. Suddenly, the cinema doors opened, and a who's who of Hollywood walked past us as we gawped like a pair of star-struck teenagers.

A tiny person with her blond hair up in a Germanic Heidi-style, arm in arm with someone I soon realised was Steven Meisel, the renowned photographer, stopped on the red carpet in front of me for a long moment and slowly looked me bitchily up and down, before continuing on.

From the screams of "Ma Daaana!" all around, I realised who it was. The crime I had committed? Wearing the same dress as her; a long, red Adidas number with a white stripe up the side. Surprisingly cheap attire for a multimillionaire superstar.

I never saw her in *that* again, but she lent it to her son David years later, who made front page headlines wearing it.

Back in the trendy lounge on 10th Street, Eddy and I were leaning on the bar, soaking up the ambience. The lights had been switched off, and there were tiny candles everywhere. John, the handsome barman, happened to be from Livingston, not far from Edinburgh. He was drawn like a magnet to Eddy. "Well, halloo," she said, her eyes undressing him. "What brings *you* to New York?"

"I shagged half of Scotland," John replied. "So I had to get oot and find a new stomping ground."

"Let me introduce myself," she said, shaking his hand firmly. "I'm Eddy. I shagged the other half!"

They started flirting o u t r a g e o u s l y with each other, and Eddy did her coy, half-turn-hair-flip, closing her eyes and laughing sexily at whatever John had just whispered in her ear.

Suddenly we all started to smell something burning. Eddy's long, red locks had touched a candle and were starting to sizzle. Quick as a flash, John chucked a bucket of ice from the bar all over her. Rather than be angry, she shrieked with laughter, and the whole place erupted in applause, very possibly because that evening, she happened to be wearing a tight T-shirt and no bra. The hot sun was coming up as the party cooled down. As usual, we realised that we'd spent all of our money and didn't have any left for a cab fare. Two girls going to a cashpoint at 6 a.m. was just asking for trouble. We cunningly developed three potential ways of getting home:

1. Chat someone up who had a car.

2. Get a cab to a bagel shop near our apartment, ask the cabbie to wait while we order, then sneak out the back and run home.

3. Hail a ride on the back of a screaming fire truck going uptown, grabbing onto the engine for dear life.

Option 3 was the one we used the most.

Working in one of the city's busiest emergency centres was unreal. You never knew what was coming next through those plastic fringed curtains that separated us from the ambulance bay. The hospital was located on swanky 5th Avenue, but at its boundary with Harlem. This made for an interesting mix of patients. An overdosed homeless hooker could be on a stretcher next to an overdosed Hollywood star.

We had a burly police officer permanently on duty, both to calm down the fights in the waiting room and to check any shady character's pockets for drug paraphernalia or weapons.

It was the middle of the AIDS epidemic, and we had to be extra careful when taking and handling blood. Sadly, several members of staff were infected just during my short time there. No real treatment existed in those days, and many people died of respiratory complications such as tuberculosis. I walked around permanently wearing a protective gown, bonnet, two pairs of gloves, an eye shield and a mask, like some kind of mad nuclear scientist.

We got to know the regulars; many were patients with drug addictions looking for methadone, the morphine substitute. They knew all the tricks. Often friendly and very funny despite their tough existence, it made me sad to imagine how low you must feel to end up like them, with their hollow faces, shrunken bodies, pinpoint pupils and scars covering their arms from needle tracks. Just a little hit of "f r e e" crack one day to make them forget the pain and desolation, only to find themselves hooked and prisoners to the pushers. Or worse, infected with HIV. One guy had abused his veins so badly that the only place I could find one to get an IV into was his penis.

We didn't even bother arguing with them after a while. If they wanted to get seen quickly, they'd just say they had chest pain; they knew that we were obliged to perform an immediate ECG and let them in. One desperate girl even set her hair on fire with a cigarette lighter in the waiting room in order to push to the front of the queue. Maybe Eddy gave her the tip-off? There were always wall-to-wall stretchers. When these were full of elderly people, a colleague remarked poetically that it was like a nursery gone full circle.

Often patients were on ventilators and very seriously ill. Managers played the eternal game of Find a Bed. Patients could stay several days in our unit, sleeping on a hard trolley, waiting to be hospitalised. This particular hospital accepted patients with Medicare and Medicaid (low-income health insurance), so it was a popular place.

This also made it a dangerously busy place. I remember having to physically clamber over three stretchers whilst clutching a heavy machine in order to defibrillate some poor soul in the corner who was having a cardiac arrest.

One night, a psychiatric patient managed to get through security with a hidden gun. After pointing it at us all, he grabbed one of the Filipino nurses, held the weapon to his hostage's head and asked him to "Sing something by Luther Vandross, or I'll kill you." As the whole room held its breath, astonishingly, the male nurse managed to stammer out the first few lines of *Never too much*.

"Ok, good," the gunman told him. "I liked that. I think I love you. Will you marry me?"

"Oh yes, I will!" answered our colleague, clasping his hands together. "I'll just pop off and call my mum in the Philippines. Tell her the good news."

As he scampered away, the patient was disarmed, handcuffed, and immediately given a powerful sedative.

People are so strange and unpredictable that we had to be prepared for anything potentially jaw-dropping. Nothing shocks a nurse! At least if it does, you mustn't show it. On another busy evening, an ambulance arrived in the bay, the paramedics pushing a stretcher towards us with a bizarre shape on it, all covered by a large, white sheet.

It turned out to be a lady in a state of vaginismus (involuntary vaginal muscle contraction) post-coitus with her dog. The poor dog was trapped. We had to administer ketamine, an anaesthetic agent, in order to release the unfortunate animal. I wish I could say it was just a little poodle, but a Saint Bernard would be closer to the mark. I did wonder about calling up the American equivalent of the RSPCA. Hopefully, karma really exists, and these people will be reincarnated as Brighton hamsters.

Animals get everywhere in New York it would seem. Many a morning, I would bite into my deli muffin/bagel, only to choke on and then spit out the remnants of a rat's tail. Yes, you read that right! Insects were especially common, too. Many of the old apartment buildings are infested with cockroaches. We had hundreds of patients arrive in the middle of the night, almost convulsing in panic. Waiting until their unsuspecting victim has gone to sleep, these little critters climb into their favourite cosy, warm place – the human ear. One is awakened suddenly by agonising scratching, which seems to originate from right inside one's brain. The only thing that can kill these vermin is neat alcohol poured directly into the inner ear via a syringe. Once they stop wriggling around, long tweezers are inserted to fish them out, an excruciatingly painful procedure, especially if the patient moves. Which, let's face it, they usually do.

I slept with earplugs after the first cockroach incident, the only downside being that I often got into trouble for getting to work late, not having heard my alarm clock go off.

One insect incident I particularly remember happened upon an unfortunate elderly gentleman who got bitten by a tick in the scrotum. A tick is an eight-legged, five mm-long parasite which feeds on blood. This one needed to be removed quickly before potentially transmitting various pathologies such as typhus and Lyme disease.

One of the ER residents thus immediately took charge of the patient; undressed him from the waist down, laid him on a stretcher in one of the cubicles, closed the curtains, popped his knees apart and started fishing around for the blood-sucking bug, closely hunched over the poor man's testicles with a pair of tweezers.

The high-pitched squeal of a disgusted "No Waaaay!" accompanied by dry heaving omitting from the secretary who opened the curtains by mistake could be heard around the entire emergency room. Possibly the whole hospital. We couldn't blame her imagination; it was an easy misinterpretation to make in that crazy place. Anything was possible. Staff were always getting caught engaging in various sexual acts in the unlikeliest of places: empty ward beds, on-call rooms, stairwells, the hospital roof, the helicopter, an operating table… there *were* even a few "stiffs" reported in the morgue!

To give another example of this New York craziness, a patient came in having had the original idea of placing a white, pink-maned My Little Pony toy into his rectum. I sat at his head, administering Entonox (laughing gas) and reassurance while the surgical registrar foraged around down below.

Ever concerned that the simple procedure may not work and he'd need a laparotomy (opening up the abdomen), I asked the doc if he was going to be OK.

She looked up at me and winked. "I'd call his condition *stable*," she replied.

Generally speaking, an RN in the States has a great deal more autonomy than an RGN in the UK. We were allowed to assess the patients in triage, decide who to see first, which blood work and X-rays or ultrasounds to order, who should get an IV or oxygen, which patients should be kept nil by mouth or who should have a gastric tube popped down their nose. Our job was basically to search for clues and go to the medical staff when we had an idea of what the crime was. It was like playing Nurse Holmes and Dr Watson.

When a patient presented with a certain problem or symptom, unless it was perfectly obvious, like a broken leg, there were a number of what we called "differential diagnoses". For example, if someone came through the door with acute pain in their right lower quadrant (we split the abdomen into four square parts - not literally you understand, just metaphorically), the immediate assumption might be that it was appendicitis, especially if the patient was young and had an accompanying low-grade fever. But that, of course, would be too easy…

• If it was a female patient of child-bearing age, we couldn't dismiss an ectopic pregnancy.
• Gall bladder stones could be the cause, particularly in an

FFFF patient (Fair, Female, Fat, Forty).

- If there was associated lower back pain in someone with cardiovascular issues, a dissecting abdominal aortic aneurysm needed to be ruled out. If *that* ruptures, the patient could die in seconds, so it's definitely better to check.
- It could also be Crohn's disease, various pelvic cysts, abscesses or hernias. Or maybe cystitis. The list goes on…

We nurses were allowed to administer certain medicines or treatments without going via the doctors (once we had proven ourselves and gained their trust). There were numerous asthma and sickle-cell anaemia sufferers in a purely nurse-led unit, using predetermined protocols, long before nurse-led units and protocols even existed in many places.

I once took a risky decision to put an external pacemaker on a cardiac patient whose heart was beating too slowly and who was about to pass out. The ER doctors were busy and the patient had bad closed-angle glaucoma, meaning that the usual treatment (IV atropine) was contraindicated. I nervously called the cardiologist to explain my decision, ready to face the firing squad because pacemaker patches are horrendously expensive and can only be used once when opened. He actually *thanked* me! If I'd dared to do that in the UK, the cardiologist would have probably spontaneously combusted, spluttering in indignant outrage.

This medical freedom didn't obliterate the caring factor, far from it. Patient contact was as important as ever. The job was, in many ways, just more recognised, appreciated and challenging. We were nurses, not doctors… and very proud of it. Eddy turned out to be one of the most knowledgeable and gifted of us all; even the top consultants came to her for advice, and the New York Times wrote an elaborate article about her work. That flame-haired party girl saved many, many lives.

Occasionally, I worked extra hours on the cardiac ICU (intensive care unit). We each had one patient. One! Leaving us free to devote ourselves completely, using everything we had learnt in giving total, delicate, research-based care. It was nursing heaven. In the UK, one ICU nurse can have five or six patients to look after.

On a daily, sometimes nightly basis, however, it remained a pretty stressful job. We were working thirteen-hour shifts, sometimes with only a quick ten-minute break for Chinese takeout and watery coffee. Neither mistakes nor death were acceptable, and those plastic fringed curtains from the ambulance bay to the ER never stopped swinging back and forth.

In America, everyone apart from the most low-income families or people with disabilities (who have Medicaid and Medicare programmes) needs to obtain a private health plan. If you consult a doctor, you are almost always required to make additional payments. The average American family spends about $1,300 per month, and not all employers help out. The USA spends more on healthcare than any other country, not only because it is so expensive but also because the population suffers high levels of chronic diseases, such as hypertension, diabetes and obesity.

Unfortunately, many people avoid seeing a doctor or dentist as a result. The waiting time in our ER could be around sixteen hours for non-emergency consultations, but people waited. They simply didn't have the means to go to a GP.

We all felt the need to get away from the mayhem sometimes and unwind. Down in Alphabet City was one of Eddy's and my favourite hangout places, a semi-legal after-hours private club bizarrely known as Save the Robots. Once we left – or got thrown out of – a normal night club, we'd often head down there afterwards.

Past the entrance and first doorman, a long flight of steps led down to a dingy, foul-smelling, dark corridor along to another windowless door through which you could feel the music thumping before actually hearing it. The second bouncer would only let you pass if you were a regular customer, famous or knew the boss personally.

Inside, it was almost pitch-black, the bar being just visible and selling one drink only: vodka. Dotted around the place were floor-to-ceiling poles meant for winding various parts of your body around in time to the beat. The air was full of smoke: a heady mixture of tobacco and hashish.

One night, we'd been dancing our socks off for a solid few hours when suddenly there was a blinding light, and someone shouted, "Freeze y'all and ass-*ume* the po-*sition*!" Save the Robots was being busted. We leant, shakily, facing the nearest wall with our hands above our heads. I was already imagining being fired, told to pack up my stuff and booted onto the next plane back to England.

As our pockets were being searched, I snuck a look at either side of me. Eddy was on my right, being rather slowly groped by a tall, dark policeman. To my left was a familiar-looking, tattooed, muscly guy with dreadlocks who winked at me with a stoned smile. Fortunately, they apparently found little of interest and we were told to vacate the premises "…*immediately, please, ma'am.*"

Walking back uptown, blinking in the hazy morning sunshine and listening out for a fire engine, it suddenly dawned on me who the guy was. It's not every day you get frisked next to Lenny Kravitz! Lyricist of *Let Love Rule* – my all-time favourite song.

Eddy dated Mark, the policeman, for a while. There didn't seem to be a man on earth who could resist her charms. She dumped him after he tried to handcuff her one night.

It had been around two years since we'd arrived in New York. Eddy had somehow found out about this "greet wee cowboy bar doon-toon", and I'd agreed to go with her to check it out. Standing outside Hogs and Heifers in the shabby meat-packing district, amongst the Harley Davidsons, pointy boots, and Stetsons, I wondered if I'd done the right thing. I'd loved my after-school country dancing classes as a kid but had never been a great fan of the thigh-slapping music and "hee-haws."

As we walked in, dressed in matching white sequin boob-tubes and McRae tartan shorts I'd had made from some material dad had given me, I noticed an interesting mixture of spit and sawdust on the floor amid hostile stares. A dreary country and western band were playing in the corner, twanging their guitars and banjos. As they finished their repertoire, the lead singer came round the bar holding out a bowl. He stopped in front of us.

"Any tips for the band, honey?" he said. "Yeah," I replied. "Don't quit your day jobs."

The bored-looking barmaid poured us each a large mojito, saying that if we could cheer the place up, they'd be on the house.

No need to ask twice, of course. Eddy jumped up on the counter, with me not far behind. We got the place alive and kicking in no time. It was suddenly full, heaving, sweaty and fun. Singing our hearts out to Joni Mitchell's *Big Yellow Taxi*, we grabbed people up onto the bar for singing, dancing and tequila shots, encouraged by the barmaid who also happened to be the owner. We must have made an impression because we were offered permanent jobs on the spot.

But, much more importantly, that night a man with cheeky green eyes and a delicious French accent actually looked past Eddy and came over to *me*. He shouted, whilst tapping his watch, "Chérie! Ze babysitter is waiting. We must go home, our little one needs feeding and changing ze nappy." The crowd around us looked horrified; this wanton hussy dancing on the table-tops was a *mother*?

I was stunned for just a moment, before realising it was a joke. I had become used to the fact that *septic tanks*[1] in my albeit short experience were generally a little humour-challenged. I decided to play along. Getting down off the bar, we clinked shot glasses and spent the entire evening pretending to be married. His name was Christophe, he was Parisian and a final-year business student at NYU. Suddenly, there were just the two of us in the room, and from that night on, I was hooked.

Before going home at dawn, after politely declining the offer of employment, we were asked by the owner to leave something as a souvenir. Without hesitation, and not for the first time, Eddy whipped off her bra. Of course, as usual, I did the same. They were ceremoniously hammered to the wall behind the bar – one a size 36C, the other 32AA. The debut of a Hogs and Heifers legend apparently, as thereafter it became something of a custom for female celebrities to do the same.

I floated back uptown with a stupid grin on my face, no longer noticing the graffiti-covered, urine-stinking subway. Christophe's mobile number was firmly pushed into the pocket of my tartan shorts. I didn't know it yet, but I'd met the person I was to marry, have two children, a home and a morbidly obese guinea pig with.

"Don't call him *too* soon; make him suffer," was Eddy's advice. "Treat 'em mean and keep 'em keen… the egg doesn't swim towards the sperm, now does it?"

I waited a whole morning before reaching for the phone.

We started dating a week later after a few flirty calls, and the smile on my face and butterflies in my tummy haven't stopped

---

[1] Cockney rhyming slang for "*Yanks*". Particularly the white male kind. Many of them seemed to have swapped their personalities for a baseball cap.

to this day. Having kissed all the princes, I ended up falling in love with a frog. Being a student, he had little money, so it was I who paid for the restaurants, ski trips to Vermont and weekends in Long Island. But I had struck human gold. He was the kindest, funniest, most generous and intelligent person I had ever met.

And by then, I'd met an awful lot of people.

We flew over to Montpellier in the south of France to meet his rather bemused parents in their *maison secondaire* (holiday house). They seemed very nice, even if they looked at me strangely. I didn't understand a word of what they were chattering on about, but I accepted their kind hospitality graciously. "My mother-in-law is lovely," he told me, "but you should know she's a maniac." After voicing my concerns about staying in a house with an axe-wielding, psychopathic serial killer, he explained that being a *maniac* in France is simply someone obsessed with tidiness.

Christophe came on my trips away with Eddy and the girls (who adored him) to Vegas, San Francisco, Miami, New Orleans and Boston. Internal travel in the States in the '90s was incredibly cheap. We headed to La Guardia or JFK on our days off, and having Irish friends who travel-nursed all over America, we generally found a sofa or an apartment floor to crash on.

Two of these girls we'd met in New York; Helena and Adele were sisters, originally from Dublin, and told us stories about some of the patients they'd met on their American travels. In Alabama, Helena had come across a lady who was convinced that God had turned her into a man at the ripe old age of eighty-four.

"I gawn an' got one of them-there penises, ma'am, strike me down if it ain't so. And it's a purdy big one, too," she'd said, chewing on a piece of black tobacco. "It is the will of our good Lord that I no longer be a woman. He sure does work in mysterious ways!" And with a guttural clearing of the throat, she expectorated something dark and frothy onto the ground in front of her feet.

Could it be true? She *did* have a bit of beard growth, thought Helena.

"Let's have a look, then. Take your underwear off, please, madam," she instructed.

As a pair of huge, grey knickers dropped to the floor, a prolapsed uterus swung down between her knees. (When pelvic ligaments are severely weakened or stretched, the uterus may fall and droop.)

Jay… sus!

"No, my dear, you're still a lady to be sure, to be sure. Just a slightly inside-out one. I'll arrange a gynaecology outpatient appointment for you immediately. You'll be just fine."

Adele then told us about a young woman living in a caravan who'd turned up at a Nashville hospital with a suspected brain haemorrhage after a fight with her trailer park neighbour. Adele accompanied her for an MRI head scan. An MRI is basically a huge, very powerful magnet. Radiology departments, therefore, have strict rules about *no metal allowed*.

"Have you ever had metal explosions in your body?" "Nope."

"Do you have any metal implants in your body?" "No, ma'am."

"Do you have any metal jewellery on your person?" "No, I sure ain't."

After the questionnaire was completed, she was taken into the radiology department and laid down on a stretcher, which was rolled into the centre of the MRI machine. Suddenly, she shot up into the air and was stuck hard to the enormous magnet suspended by her breasts, cursing and screaming for help.

Wearing an underwired bra can be a dangerous thing! You've been warned, ladies.

I had discovered a lifelong passion for travelling. I got such a buzz out of this nomadic lifestyle. America was an amazing place to start: the breath-taking Grand Canyon, the gorgeous beaches at Carmel, and the blue forests of New England in autumn… it is a truly magnificent country.

The only thing is that the further away you get from New York, the higher the religious fanatic factor rises. The radio is a great measuring instrument for this. NYC music stations play pop, rock and jazz, which gradually change into country and western songs about God, guns, trucks and hillbilly hand-fishing the further south or west you go. Non-redneck music comes back on around fifty miles east of San Francisco.

We had a few strange religious folk visit the ER at times. A lady came in one day, looking as white as a sheet, clutching her lower left quadrant, accompanied by her husband. The echography, unfortunately, showed that she had an ectopic pregnancy. This is where the foetus starts to develop in one of the fallopian tubes instead of the uterus. If this ruptures, the resulting bleeding can kill the mother. The only solution is emergency surgery.

"Do you know if your wife has a blood-type card, please?" I asked the husband gently while she was behind the curtains being prepped for theatre.

"Oh no," he replied, "we're Jehovah's Witnesses, and my wife will not be having a transfusion; I forbid it."

"But, sir, she may not survive without it!"

"I don't care. Blood contains Satan."

What the…?! This was a new one on me.

I beeped our senior on-call anaesthesiologist. He explained to me that certain cell-saver transfusion methods exist, which economise the bags of blood and frozen plasma that we normally give during surgical procedures. Instead, the blood that is directly lost from the patient can be washed, centrifuged and given back if necessary. Would she be willing to accept this?

As a matter of fact, luckily, it turned out that her husband would.

I respect religious beliefs, but to me, this was verging on misogynistic domestic violence. As I held out the insurance forms for the husband to sign, I believe he could read the contempt in my eyes. Surely this decision was not his to make?

"I don't care what anybody thinks," he declared. "Jesus loves me!"

Maybe so, I thought. But personally… *I think you're a bit of a twat.*

Unlike Satan, New York gets into your blood… but slowly my Frenchman found his way into my heart and got lodged there for good. Christophe had finished his studies at NYU and had a job offer in Paris. He asked me to go with him.

Eddy and I were like sisters after three crazy years together, sharing an apartment, all our favourite clothes, darkest secrets and fake tan. I was earning good money and enjoying my job, despite the depressingly endless cycle of gang revenge stabbing and gunshot wounds (their deaths only made one person happy: the organ donor coordinator). But the thought of letting Christophe go to Paris without me was inconceivable.

Saying goodbye to Eddy was the hardest part. I knew she'd survive fine without me, but she was one in a million, and I'd miss her as much as I'd miss rollerblading in the park, coffee shop capers in Union Square, open-air concerts up at Jones Beach, scrounging drinks off rich businessmen at the Windows on the World bar in the Twin Towers, the endless sirens, Reese's peanut butter ice cream and all-you-can-eat-sushi for twenty dollars.

If the world has a pulse, you'll find it in NYC. There's never a dull moment nor a time when you can say you've seen and done it all. It's fun, busy, smelly and insane, blazing hot in summer and freezing cold in winter. But it's where everyone can just be themselves.

Walk around wearing nothing but a live python and stilettos, and no one will blink an eye. Madonna famously once roamed around the East Village naked under a see-through raincoat, and nobody noticed! Hooded drug dealers mingle happily with striped-shirted Wall Street types down in Greenwich. A famous Kennedy hails a yellow cab on Park Avenue while a jogger runs past. Bagel, pretzel, and coffee booths waft delicious aromas on every corner.

Police ride their horses from Battery Park right up 5th Avenue, never distracted by the honking traffic or teenage skaters weaving between the cars. Wannabe actors work in bars and restaurants, patiently dreaming of being discovered and stardom. Homeless people, clutching Styrofoam cups with fingerless gloves, crouch for warmth over the smoking subway grills when the weather turns bad. Women working the perfume counters in Macy's and Bloomingdale's fight each other to shower you in a misty cloud of their wares as soon as you come near. On a sunny day, the blue sky reflects off the millions of little skyscraper windows as well as the Hudson and East rivers, turning Manhattan into a sparkling island jewel. At night during the Christmas season, the trees in Central Park glitter with thousands of twinkling fairy lights.

There are sights and sounds and smells you can't get anywhere else. You can find any kind of food, listen to any kind of music and cross paths with personalities of all colours, races, backgrounds and religions 24-7-365.

New York had become, and still is, my absolute favourite city on earth. It was a wrench to leave, not least because I couldn't speak any French. Christophe said he would teach me.

"Don't worry, eet's not difficult, everyone speaks Hinglish, not a problem…" He would eat his words as I'd choke on mine. I'd obtained a pitiful D grade in O-level German, so to say I was linguistically challenged would be an understatement. But when you're twenty-five, in love and off to the world's most romantic city, a certain optimism kicks in. At least at the beginning.

My leaving party at work was in the middle of a night shift in the ER, with a banquet of our favourite Golden Garden Chinese takeaway boxes and a few bottles of dishwater the Americans call beer. The public faith in medical staff not to partake in substance abuse while at work conveniently covers all manner of sins by all manner of health professionals. The party was interrupted at 3 a.m. by one of the usual local drunks who'd got himself stabbed – again. This time it was pretty serious; he was losing a lot of blood. We all rushed into action, hooking up a transfusion, using the little that was left of our precious O-negative stock whilst compressing, cleaning, and then sewing up the wound.

I was standing beside the drunken, disorientated patient on his stretcher, squeezing the bag with all my force in order to pass those vital red cells as quickly as possible into his bloodstream. All of a sudden, I felt a warm sensation over my legs. I looked down at a toothless smile as I realised that I was being used as the proverbial tree by the proverbial dog.

Since working in the ER, I'd now been pissed on, slapped, scratched, farted at, spat on, puked over, kicked, verbally insulted, threatened and had both HIV-positive blood and faeces thrown in my face.

"Well," I said to myself, "things can't possibly get worse than this where I'm going."

And in the end, I didn't have to worry about Eddy. Standing at a crossroads in Tribeca one afternoon in May, a large, powerful motorbike purred up to the red light she was waiting at. The rider opened his visor to get a proper and very appreciative look at my old flatmate. The appreciation was mutual, and Eddy being Eddy, accepted his offer of a spare helmet and straddled the bike behind him. They rode down Broadway and off into the sunset. Eddy and George married a year later in the Hamptons.

She also went on to become the new hospital director.

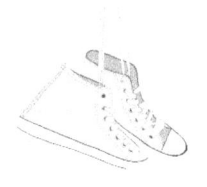

4. PARIS

Real friends and faux pas

Arriving jet-lagged at Charles de Gaulle airport early one morning, the place looked like a space station in a cheap sci-fi film. All glass lifts, escalators and walkways crossing over each other. The first thing I noticed was that *everyone* was smoking. We walked outside to hail a cab, kicking through orange cigarette butts like fallen leaves in autumn.

Climbing out of the airport taxi in central Paris, the air rising up from the cobbled streets was warm and humid from a recent rainstorm. I was still a bit shaky from the ride. Not yet used to Parisian driving, both my knuckles and hair had turned white whilst our driver negotiated the infamous Place de l'Etoile under the Arc de Triomphe. I had actually made the sign of the cross, despite being agnostic, sure that we were about to live our last seconds. The basic idea is to get into the centre of this huge roundabout and drive so fast that you can exit without difficulty, whatever vehicle may be hurtling towards your right side at the speed of light. Amazingly, accidents there are rare.

We were renting a small, poky apartment belonging to Christophe's aunt. The rent was cheap in exchange for looking after her precious *Chaussette* (Sock), thus named as it had three white paws and one black one. He was a malicious, devious tabby. Whenever the feline fiend didn't get his *croquettes* (biscuits) on demand, he left us a squishy brown reminder outside our bedroom door. I hated that animal and vice versa. All I wanted to do was kick it up the backside and use it *as* a sock.

Christophe enjoyed showing me all his favourite places. We ambled around Montmartre hand in hand, winding in and out of the street artists, visited the magical Egyptian treasures in the Louvre and made the exhausting climb to the top of the Eiffel Tower in order to avoid paying the extortionate price for the lift.

We walked through every park, visited every museum and even ventured underground into the murky, skull-filled catacombs. Crossing the bridges over the Seine, we'd throw scrunched-up balls of tissue paper onto the heads of Japanese tourists sitting in rows below on the Bateaux Mouches, ducking out of view like a pair of naughty teenagers.

We drank overpriced coffee at Les Deux Maggots pretending to be Jean-Paul Sartre and Simone de Beauvoir. We sipped overpriced Côtes du Rhône at the plush Hôtel Costes in St- Germain-des-Près. We hung out on café terrasses, drinking in the odour of expressos and buttery *pain-au-chocolats*. And in the bars of Le Marais, I attempted to join in with the sweaty locals, dancing *La Salsa, Le Tango* and *Le Rock.*

We embarked on a day trip to Disneyland, returning home a sickly shade of grey after going on the Tower of Terror three times and eating too much *barbe à papa* (candy floss). I gawped in awe at the magnificent Galerie des Glaces, spectacular fountains and mirrored gardens of the Palace of Versailles. We meandered around the gorgeous pink Petit Trianon, where badass Marie-Antoinette hung out and partied such a long time ago. I wondered if Eddy might somehow be related to her.

As we sat on the steps of the Sacré-Cœur church snuggling up together one evening, overlooking the rooftops of Paris, watching the July shooting stars, dreaming, planning and making wishes, I knew I had made the right decision to come here.

A month later, still a little dizzy from restless, eerily quiet, siren-free nights, I had a CDD (limited-time French employment contract) at St Emilion's hospital in Paris' 5th district. Only in France could a hospital be named after a wine region.

I'd posted my CV upon arrival to all the hospitals in our area and struck lucky. It was the middle of summer. Paris was hot, airless and sticky. The city's hospital beds were full but understaffed. Parisian healthcare workers were off sunning themselves on the Côte d'Azur or in Corsica, alongside the ones who'd already had their holidays and were now on strike or curiously *malade* (ill). France quite simply comes to a halt for the summer months.

Luckily, British nursing diplomas are recognised throughout much of Europe, unlike in the States, where I'd had to sit an exam. And by another stroke of luck, no language test was organised. Even if you're a swan-eating Old Etonian with ten plums in your mouth, you still need to pass a basic English test in order to nurse in America.

I was, however, required to validate my nursing certificate at the *préfecture* in Nanterre, on the outskirts of Paris. I made my way to arrive at the arranged appointment time on the RER (Paris' combined city-centre underground and suburban commuter rail system) with all the necessary documents triple-checked in hand. In front of the main gates was a large board informing the public which floor to go to for which service.

Floor eighteen was for *Affaires Sanitaires et Sociales*. I checked this was the right department noted on my piece of paper from HR, then hit the button for the lift. Stepping out at the eighteenth floor, I followed the corridor round to a desk marked *Certificats et Diplômes*, sitting behind which was a typically obnoxious-looking *fonctionnaire,* as French state workers are known.

This beady-eyed, long-faced guy resembled a bored rat. I stood there for five minutes waiting for him to acknowledge me, but he didn't look up from his computer screen. I cleared my throat.

"*Bonjour monsieur.* Can you help me, *s'il vous plaît?*" I said, putting on my most charming, endearing, wide-eyed smile. Without his stamp, I couldn't get a job. And he damn well knew it.

His radar immediately picked up my English accent. I could almost read his mind deciding whether or not to use the power he had over me to rip my employment ambitions to shreds. He sighed unnecessarily loudly and, at last, favoured me with a stony glance. Looking at his watch, it was 11.45 a.m., he dismissed me with a hand flick.

"*On est fermé.*"

Shit. "But monsieur, it says you close at midday… *Vous fermez à midi, non?*"

Another monumental sigh, eyes turned heavenwards. Regret swept over me that I hadn't gotten up earlier to take the 9.30 train. I started to panic. I needed that flipping stamp!

"*S' il vous plaît* – please. I have come a long way – *une heure et demie. Je dois travailler ce soir!*" I must go to work this evening, I begged him. This is, in fact, the reaction that they're after. He was lapping it up.

If I'd acted arrogant, nonchalant and sour-lipped, I'd probably immediately have received what I went there for. As it was, he told me glacially to come back after lunch. Then he closed his computer, shook on his jacket and buggered off, scowling. I'm sure I heard him murmur the word "*rosbif*" as he left.

I pondered on this as I ate my *sandwich au fromage* in the *préfecture* garden. The French, I had already been told numerous times, hate three things:

1. Apologies (they just don't get the principal)
2. Waiting in line (why should they?)
3. Exaggeration (apart from the inhabitants of Marseille, who live by it)

If you have the misfortune to over or under-judge something, they'll huff and puff and blow "*Faut pas exagérer!*" all over you.

We Brits use two words more than any other: sorry and please. We also have a tendency to feel guilty, be humble, queue up and get out of the way. None of this does you any good in France. *Au contraire!* As the church bells chimed at 2 p.m., I decided to head back in, using a different tactic.

Walking up to ratman, I put on my rudest face. No *bonjour* this time, "*Alors, maintenant ça suffit!* I start my new job in a few hours. Where do I get my document stamped?"

Looking slightly perplexed and rather surprised, he simply answered, "*16ème étage, madame.*"

"*Et voilà!*" I said cheekily. "*Quand vous voulez, eh?*" You see, you can when you try.

Turning my back before he could retort, I skipped down the two flights of stairs to the sixteenth floor. It was totally quiet. There wasn't a hint of life. I double-checked the floor – sixteen – before inspecting every room; all were empty, apart from a few scattered cardboard boxes. It was as if this entire floor had been hurriedly deserted due to some toxic virus. I was starting to get the creeps.

Just as I was about to flee for the lift and get the hell out, I heard a slight cough. It seemed to have come from behind one of the desks. I tiptoed over and peered behind the nearest one. A wrinkly face peered back up, scaring the life out of me.

"B… *bonjour monsieur… je, je cherche* a stamp? *Pour* my nurse, er, *infirmière diplôme. Je suis*, er, *Anglaise*. English," I stammered.

"*17ème étage,*" he said in a croaky voice, gesturing towards the elevator.

I looked around me for the hidden camera… this had to be a joke. The 17th floor? "*Vous êtes sûre?*"

"*Oui oui,*" he said, nodding, seeming indeed very sure of himself. "Nomber siventen for ze ingleesh norsees."

OK then. Back up one floor, I scampered. He was right; the busy health department was indeed on floor seventeen. I got my documents stamped by another snooty *fonctionnaire*, but without any further hitch. As I was about to leave, I went to the front desk on the ground floor.

"*Excusez-moi*. Why is it marked floor number eighteen for health matters when it's actually seventeen, but you have to go via the *sixteenth* floor?" I asked curiously.

"Ah!" replied the administrative assistant, waving her hands dismissively. "Zis way more employees 'ave got something to do."

Un – believable. *Bienvenue* to the French administrative system.

The recruiting department at St Emilion's had put me on night shifts, obviously hoping I'd have no conversations with their patients, what with them being asleep. Logically, this way I'd make fewer balls-ups which could potentially get *them* into trouble.

I arrived early to get my badge and was given three spanking clean uniforms. I started the rounds at 7 p.m. after the handover. It was a cardiology ward, and I was doubled with a very friendly and even more forgiving colleague, Estelle. We visited each patient, gave them their medication, took their "obs", and settled them in for the night.

All was going swimmingly until we entered the room of Madame Legrand, a ninety-year-old lady admitted the previous evening for congestive heart failure. Poor Madame Legrand had seen better days. She didn't respond to our voices, neither to my prodding, gentle shaking or Estelle's slapping. I had never before seen a nurse slap a patient and was justifiably shocked, even if it was a very gentle one. But my new co-worker assured me that in France, it was *normale*.

You must remember that I had spent the past few years working in a country where human life is absolutely sacred, whatever the age, and saving it is of the utmost importance, whatever the illness. Sometimes, actors had been wheeled into the ER in New York, pretending to be patients; hospital evaluation policy. Making the slightest mistake, even on an actor, could cost you your job. I don't think it's such a bad idea; it kept us on our toes, anyway.

American patients' relatives wrote down our names and photographed everything we did. We were taught to preserve life, to do absolutely everything possible in order to avoid the unthinkable. Not on *my* shift! There was no such thing as DNR on a chart (Do Not Resuscitate).

Each time an ambulance arrived, it was followed by at least three cars carrying lawyers, all watching and waiting to see if anyone had the misfortune to die. Leaving their *other* fortunes for these sharks to squabble over, often ruining nursing and medical careers in the process. If you lost someone's life in a US hospital, you could very well spend the rest of *yours* dressed in an orange jumpsuit peering through a barred window.

With this in mind, having searched Madame Legrand in vain for signs of breathing or a pulse, I ran as fast as my legs would carry me in the direction of the defibrillator. The emergency trolley crashed through the door to the patient's room with me hot on its heels. I charged the paddles up to 200 joules with a long beep, ready to administer the lifesaving electricity.

But Estelle was having none of it – she threw her hands up in horror, pushed my arms away from the patient's chest and closed Madame Legrand's eyes. I stared at her, uncomprehending – was I in the presence of an assassin? Did she actually *want* the patient to die? Wasn't that against every human ethic and professional conduct that I had learnt over the past years?

Estelle looked at me and said slowly in pidgin English, "Let zis old laydee go in peace. We must make her look nice now for ze familee."

It was then that I realised France and America were not only separated by an ocean. French nursing students are taught that phrase made famous by Ghandi: "*On juge la grandeur d'une nation à la façon dont ses faibles sont traités.*" In essence, the greatness of a nation may be judged by the way it treats its weakest. This was a whole new way of looking at things.

Crashing up and down on this lady's chest, possibly breaking a few ribs in the process, toasting her with electricity and shoving a tube down her throat without anaesthesia probably wasn't really the kindest thing to do, I had to agree. Especially as her life expectancy afterwards probably wouldn't be long or particularly pleasant. It was the final page of a unique and beautiful ninety-year-old story and time to gently close the book.

Estelle and I bonded over a cup of tea in the staff room, our PG

Tips slightly salty from tears. We've been close ever since. She told me about the job she had before arriving there in an EHPAD, a medicalised retirement home. It was like listening to a horror story. The elderly patients were so badly treated it defied belief. She said that staffing was minimised to a point where bed baths could only be given once a week, and even then, it was just a quick wipe of the bottom and armpits (hopefully not in that order). And incontinence pads were rationed to three per day per resident.

She showed me photos she'd discretely taken of people being dragged out of bed by their hair, completely ignored by "*la direction*". Breakfast, she told me, consisted of mashing up bread, butter, jam, coffee granules, orange juice and medication into a bowl together. The bowl was left for an hour in front of each person and cleared up afterwards. If they hadn't eaten anything, which most of them couldn't manage to do on their own and probably wouldn't want to anyway, well... too bad.

I understood now why Estelle was so against unnecessarily and cruelly prolonging the life of Madame Legrand. Thanks to her perseverance and evidence, that place eventually got closed down. She'll never work in an EHPAD again, though.

Estelle is someone who was born to nurse. She's the definition of kindness, a real-life angel. I'm truly lucky to have had her as my mentor and to be able to call her my friend.

It was when I started working at St Emilion's hospital that I really understood the extent of the smoking culture in France. Patients were allowed to smoke in their beds! The risk of oxygen igniting, causing explosions, destruction and death, didn't seem to bother anyone. Some nicotine-saturated surgeons even smoked non-filter Gitanes whilst operating. It wasn't only ciggies that were encouraged in the hospital. During the evening ward round, a large glass of sherry or two was also available – on medical prescription. I was told that this was to improve patients' appetites and help them sleep well. At least this way, they were less likely to annoy the night staff. Quite a clever idea, really.

At the time, smoking in France was permitted in bars, restaurants and on public transport, as well as in hospitals. Even for a smoker, being in a cloudy bar was an eye-watering, cough-inducing, clothes-reeking experience. Smoke wasn't the only form of socially accepted pollution, either. A major problem for someone British living in France is their music. The very *definition* of noise pollution. Jean Jacques, Serge and Claude François were names beforehand unheard of, but whose warbling voices arrived via speakers and airways with such regularity that they infected my brain and became a torturous part of my daily life. The French love their music. For us Brits, it feels like a machine-gun assault on one's ears. The most painful are birthday or wedding *soirées*, where they all dance around like happy zombies for hours on end to mind-blowingly dreadful *its* (hits) such as *Alexandrie Alexandra*, *Quand la Musique est Bonne* and *Femme*. The strangest part of the evening is when a song called *Ça Plane Pour Moi*, by the oddly named Plastic Bertrand, comes on. They all go completely insane at this point, jumping around the place like escaped lunatics on speed. Mercifully, radio DJs play the odd record from musically civilised countries such as Great Britain. At this point, you can either turn the sound back up on the radio or take your fingers out of your ears.

What they lack in musical talent, however, they make up for in cuisine. After a life of surviving on egg and chips, beans on toast and baked potatoes, I was in for a treat. The French can take the strangest ingredient and make it taste *incredible.*

A snail, for example, is basically a chewy, dry old piece of blu-tac. Until you drown it with salt, then stuff it back in its shell with herbs, butter, a little garlic, and… *voilà!* Delicious! Why they don't do the same thing with juicier earthworms or slugs, I don't know. They haven't thought of it yet, perhaps.

Despite having access to such culinary delights, nothing made my mouth water more than friends or family opening their suitcases to reveal gifts of Angel Delight, Stilton, Marmite or prawn cocktail crisps. I still haven't tasted anything in France that equals Marmite, even in their fancy Michelin-star restaurants. Christophe's face screwed up like a used tissue when he first tasted it; he looked as if he was about to throw up. I *may* have spread it on the toast a little too thickly for an amateur.

"*C'est affreux*! It's 'orrible! What the hell is this stuff made of? Petrol mixed with roadkill and *merde*?"

He did concede, albeit in a mildly begrudging fashion, that Stilton was one of the finest cheeses he'd ever tasted. All the while insisting that "Ze only posseebol explanation has to be ze Huguenots." These were the Protestants forced into exile from France during the sixteenth century, who, according to Christophe, brought their cheese-making skills over the Channel with them.

The French celebrate food rather than just simply eat it. They look down their noses at us Brits and our *dégueulasse* (disgusting) excuse for meals. In their minds, the only decent thing you can get to eat in the UK is a curry. And that's not even really English.

"The only other nation that comes close to being as good as us at cooking are the Italians," I was told regularly.

It's rather ironic, therefore, that they claim to have invented some of our most humble British dishes. They call one of these *La Raclette* and make a huge fuss with the preparation; each person has their own triangular spoon to heat up pieces of sliced *fromage* on a special contraption placed at the centre of the table before drooling it gently over their roasted *pommes de terre*. Baked potatoes and cheese, then. Hmmm… not exactly what I'd request as a last meal before execution. Reminds me of my poor student days.

Notwithstanding the image they like to portray, the truth is that they stuff their kids full of white bread and Nutella in the morning and absolutely *love* McDonald's, one of which you can find on every roundabout and in every shopping centre in the country.

The French talk about food all the time, especially when they're eating it. The main topic of conversation at lunch is what everybody would like for dinner. Quite annoying at first, but eventually, you get used to it and even find yourself joining in.

Proust, one of the country's most famous authors, dedicates an entire scene of his lifetime's work, *Remembrance of Things Past*, to painstakingly describing the taste of a shell-shaped pastry called a *madeleine* that he used to eat as a child and the memories it evoked. Only the French could get so powerfully emotional about what is essentially a small sponge cake.

And the wine! *Le vin français… oh là là!* They do know their grapes, I have to hand it to them. Liquid nectar in almost every bottle. The sugary concoctions we consumed in New York in goldfish-bowl quantities would be considered poisonous in Paris. If you dared to turn up at a posh dinner party with a bottle of Californian Chardonnay, it would more than likely end up chucked down *la toilette*.

Christophe taught me the arrogant French way of swilling, sniffing, slurping and savouring the delights of a chilled, mineral Condrieu or a deep, fruity Côte Rôtie. My dead taste buds started to come to life. Hallelujah! Praise be to Bacchus! The only thing was that I liked it a little *too* much. My friend Nicolas started calling me "Swellen" (meaning Sue Ellen, the infamous drunk character in the '80s TV show *Dallas*.) Funny. But slightly worrying at the same time…

Adele and Helena, who I'd met in New York, came over from Ireland to visit very soon after we moved to Paris. We thirsty girls went searching through the cupboards one evening for something to drink for an *apéritif* and found Christophe's hidden stash. Opening a bottle, we each poured ourselves a glass and were glugging the stuff back when he arrived home from work.

"Pour me a glass too, chérie," he said. "I've had a tough day…"

As soon as he took a sip, I immediately knew something was amiss.

"But zis is delicious!" he exclaimed with an amazed look. "Elixir from ze gods. A liquid orgasm… Amazing! My goodness. So, tell me where you bought it. I'll order a crate."

Three pairs of eyes looked down at the floorboards. "We um…

found it… in your wine cupboard."

He went insane. We'd just gulped down a bottle of 1967 Château Latour… worth about 500 euros. He'd been given it by his grandfather for his 21st birthday. We walked around sheepishly with our tails between our legs for the rest of the weekend, trying not to laugh.

"An act of gastronomic culture to us is just an alcoholic impulse to you people," huffed Christophe disdainfully. "Bunch of bloody British barbarians!" He got over it, eventually.

The *people* were much, much trickier to get used to than the food, culture, accents or even the music. Women were supposed to be ladylike – no burping, drinking or farting. And certainly no effing and blinding. So, obviously, I was off to a bad start. I'd been dragged rather than brought up, you must remember. Christophe's best friend's lovely wife actually took pity on me: tying pastel-coloured jumpers round my neck, taking me for a manicure and even buying me a Longchamp bag to replace my old, weathered back-pack in order to try and help me "*feet* in".

I nearly caused a diplomatic incident by flatly refusing to wear the fur coat and Hermès scarf that my future parents-in-law had offered me. I'm a jeans, T-shirt and Converse girl. That didn't go down well *at all*. Parisian women eat and drink next to nothing, smoke continuously, have perfect nails, and perfect figures, wear fur and fancy handbags during the day and lacy negligées at night. As a rude-joke-telling, pyjama-wearing, wine-swigging, crisp-munching, anti-fur activist, I wasn't doing much to improve the image of my fellow countrywomen.

After we'd all known each other a while, one of Christophe's friends told me, with a thoughtful expression on his face, "In an ideal world, I would marry a French girl – they are serious mothers, have beautiful figures and cook really well. But for the *maitresse* (mistress), I would choose English. So much more fun." I couldn't decide whether to hug him or slap him. So I did both.

I read somewhere that the Inuits are immune to cold, the Africans to heat and the British to irony. The French are immune… to *other people*. If your neighbour, bank clerk, waiter or shop assistant feels like pretending you're just not there, they will. The nicer you are, the worse it gets. I sincerely started to worry I'd turned invisible once, a victim of some kind of Gallic curse, whilst waiting patiently at a Renault dealers' office in the 5ème arrondissement. Nobody acknowledged me! I just snuck out when they turned the lights off.

Queueing as we know it simply doesn't exist in France. I imagine it's not taught at school, along with opening doors for others, stopping at red lights or smiling cheerfully at a stranger. This lack of waiting in an orderly fashion is most evident when attempting to embark on a ski chair lift, sitting in your car at a *péage* (motorway toll booth) or in an emergency room waiting area. The wonderful American concept of ER triage (where the most severely ill are seen in priority) goes right out the nearest window, along with all the cigarette ends. In French *urgences*, it's the one who complains the loudest who is seen first.

The more time I spent in France, the more talented I became at mimicking their gestures. My favourite is taking a deep breath and then pushing air really hard out of my cheeks through pursed lips, making a blowing-off sound. You then shrug, pout and simultaneously raise your eyes and palms. This basically conveys the message to the person opposite you that they're a mindless idiot. A simple "*Pffff*" is just as effective when you're in a hurry.

Rapidly sticking your index finger into one blown-out cheek five or six times means the person opposite you is lying or exaggerating. The French don't like exaggeration. Except for the ones who live in Marseille, as I said.

There are also some great sayings. To not give a damn is: *S'en bat les couilles*. (To knock your balls one against the other.) An interesting image. When they *really* don't want to do something, they say: "*Ça me trou le cul.*" (Literally, "That's making a hole in my arse.") Why? When there's one already. The mind boggles.

Despite being allies on the winning side during two world wars, the French dislike the English with a passion. The Scots and Irish are tolerated, having a longstanding arch-enemy in common. I personally found it extremely difficult to integrate and be accepted for a *very* long time. The first doctor I worked with in Paris casually mentioned, as if talking about the weather, that it was such a shame that the *peste* (bubonic black plague during the Middle Ages) hadn't killed us Brits all off.

The new people I met all greeted me with *la bise*, that amiable air-cheek "mwah mwah" kiss, but at the same time with a judgemental up-and-down look, which immediately made me feel like something which had just crawled out from underneath a particularly nasty cowpat.

"*Enchantée! Ah, vous êtes Anglaise… hmmm.*"

I find it strange then, to learn that, until recently, London was Frances's sixth biggest city, housing more French nationals than Bordeaux.

When I ask the inevitable question, why all the hatred? They mumble something about us killing Joan of Arc. I always ungraciously reply, "Well, you killed Princess Diana, so we're quits."[2]

There's a story I couldn't help telling at dinner parties with Christophe's anti-English friends and family, despite risking death by strangulation: "God created the world in six days, the Bible tells us. What it omitted to mention is that on the seventh day He decided to create His *chef d'oeuvre*, His masterpiece, His *pièce de*

---

[2] The rumour in medical circles has it that if the SAMU (the French emergency ambulatory service) had brought Princess Diana to the operating theatre within *the golden hour* instead of taking time trying to stabilise her in the ambulance under the Pont d'Alma, she may have survived. Sadly, we'll never know. Obviously the drunk, speeding chauffeur and the paparazzi need to take their part of the blame too. But it remains to this day a subject of intense interest and debate in France. I later worked in the SAMU and have nothing but the greatest respect for them, despite the never-ending discussion on this subject.

résistance: a land where there is a wonderful temperate climate, utterly spectacular and perfectly varied scenery, all that grows in the fertile ground there being delicious to eat. Or drink.

He named this fine land "La France!"

At this point, my French audience all nod their heads, clap and murmur in agreement.

But then, I add, "Suddenly, God slapped Himself on the forehead!"

"What have I done?" He wailed. "Now that this terrestrial paradise exists, every human will come *here*! It will become too overcrowded! No one will live in Japan, Africa, Norway or America. What shall I do to stop everybody wanting to live in France?"

And that's when He had His brilliant idea.

He created the French…

The World Health Organisation regularly votes for France as providing the best overall healthcare in the world. Around 80% of the costs are government funded, and about the same percentage is refunded to patients, who often have to pay up first, using a sort of credit card called *la Carte Vitale*. The premium is automatically deducted from employees' pay.

There are public, private and non-profit privatised hospitals. Anyone is eligible for social security after having spent at least three months in the country. As in the UK, GPs are the gatekeepers. However, anyone is free to consult a specialist at their own cost.

It's twenty-five euros to visit your designated doctor, who guarantees seeing you that same day (and is chosen by you), with about eighteen euros of this refunded. Waiting times are much shorter in general than in Great Britain, especially for elective surgical procedures.

At the time of writing, a nurse's salary averages the equivalent of around 31,000 pounds per annum. Pitiful! Further training is offered via a *concours* or competition, for paediatrics, management, theatres or anaesthesia. Nurses with specialist training can earn more.

Salaries generally increase slowly with time.

As well as their more lenient attitude towards death and smoking, one other fundamental difference between us and *les français* is their obsession with suppositories. For all age groups, the anus is the preferred passage for every possible medicine and medical instrument.

The anguished shrieks of one nurse manager is something I shall never forget, as she walked onto the ward one morning, only to find all of my patients sitting up in bed with their rectal glass thermometers stuck in their mouths. In my defence, how could I possibly have known?

During one ward medication round (where we pop the patients' pills in front of them to take with a glass of water/wine), we came back to check that Monsieur Borel, a post-cholecystectomy patient, had swallowed his. Some patients need help or simply forget. Monsieur Borel scrunched up his face in disgust at the memory of it.

"Your medicament – eet was *not* good!" he spat. My colleague checked the drug chart and immediately understood why… she burst out laughing. He'd eaten his suppository. I had thought that the pill looked a bit strange, but I just put it alongside the others without a second thought. I'd never seen a suppository before.

My biggest handicap was, of course, the language. My cockney cerebrum was very slow in soaking it up. I'd even had a hard time in New York, where they're supposed to speak English. They pronounce tuna, *toonah* and, coffee, *kwouffee,* for example. A *fanny* is a bottom, and *pants* are trousers; it's all very strange.

American patients often used to say, "I just luurve your British axe-ent."

To which I'd reply, "I don't have one, mate… you do."

When I heard people talking on the ward in Paris, it sounded like a mixture of Swedish, ancient Greek and Jabba the Hutt from Star

Wars to me. I kept my ears constantly peeled, trying to pick up the basics. Some French words sounded similar but had such a different meaning. They called them *faux amis* or false friends.

"It's the same for us!" Christophe told me. Apparently, it's impossible for them to hear the difference between sheep and ship. Or sheet and shit, for that matter.

One night in the cardiology unit, I was instructed to lie a patient flat on his stretcher in order to perform an electrocardiogram. This involves sticking several patches onto the patient's chest. For some strange reason, the French use the verb *attacher* for applying the sticky electrodes… which can also mean to tie up. And, instead of saying *baisser* (to lower), I mistakenly omitted one little *s* and pronounced it *baiser,* which literally means to shag (excuse my French).

So, whereas what I wanted to say was, "I am going to lower you down flat, sir, so that I can stick these patches on you…", what I *actually* told the patient was that I wanted to tie him up and shag him. I've never in my life seen someone look so pleasantly surprised.

"I'm so glad I took zat expensive health insurance!" he exclaimed with a satisfied smirk.

After lowering someone down on their stretcher had got me into trouble, putting them back upright didn't fare me any better. The verb to climb or go upwards in French is *monter*. But of course, that's not all it means. I must have told a hundred or so bemused patients that I was going to *mount* them before some kind soul corrected me.

It was the same problem with heat up: *chauffer*. This verb comes from the word *chaud* (warm). Whenever I put a blanket on a patient, I told them I was going to *chauffer* them. It took months of perplexed looks and stifled laughter before someone eventually told me what I should be saying when referring to a person was *rechauffer* or re-warm them. To *chauffer* someone means to get them hot and horny.

Some French words are spelt exactly the same but mean something completely different. *Allonger,* for example, is a verb meaning to stretch out flat, like your legs on the couch, whilst watching TV. But it can also mean making something longer. My male patient, in this case, was being prepped for surgery and needed to lie flat on the stretcher. I decided to avoid the dangerous word *baisser a*nd try something new.

"I'm just going to *allonger* you," I informed him.

His eyes shot wide open, like the headlights on a Porsche. "Really!" came the happy reply. "By how many centimetres?"

You can see my dilemma; no matter how hard I tried, there was always an opportunity to make a *faux pas* coupled, inevitably, with making a complete fool of myself.

Christophe was living up to his promise and helping to teach me French, but he spoke mostly *argot* or slang. I listened to him and his friends talking about women, not referring to them as *femmes* but as *meufs*, *gonzesses*, *nanas* or *pouffes*. When I later met Christophe's father, surprised to find him alone, I inquired on the whereabouts of his *pouffe*. As soon as I saw his shocked face, I knew I'd made a blunder. I'd asked my future father-in-law where his bitch was.

I got my own back when I introduced Christophe to my own father's new bride, whispering to him that her nick-name was "trouble and strife", the cockney slang for wife. That got him in well-deserved trouble.

Some of the language was easy to grasp. I noticed that the French put the word *normalement* into a sentence at every opportunity. It's strange because "normally" isn't really a word we Brits, well, normally use. I worked out that it's just an excuse not to take responsibility for anything that they might potentially be wrong about.

"We'll be there for dinner at eight sharp tonight… *normalement.*"

"*Normalement,* you'll receive the cheque within the next 48 hours."

"There are no red-hot chillies in that sauce. *Normalement.*"

"Uh-oh, those condoms were out of date. But *normalement* you'll be fine…"

After having worked there for a while, I started to get the hang of the general organisation of the cardiology ward, along with the basic types of treatment and medicine. My spoken and written French slowly but surely improved. However, that still didn't stop the odd slip-up from happening.

I had been transferred to A&E for the day to help out. A lady came in with a straightforward fractured ankle. We plastered up her leg, gave her pain killers, wrote the necessary prescriptions, and she was free to go. She became extremely distressed, however, at not being able to contact her husband to come and pick her up. I wanted to reassure her and decided to practise my novice grasp of the language.

"Don't worry, madame," said I, clearing my throat, "*Votre mari est sûrement* (your husband is surely) *en rûte.*"

What I'd wanted to say was the very similar "*en route*" (on the road or on his way). Unfortunately, *rûte* means to rut, as a large male animal on heat may spectacularly demonstrate when confronted with the female of its species during mating season.

She did not look amused… unlike the rest of the room.

Another time I came in late for work, having had car trouble. The battery was flat. After a kindly neighbour had helped me to recharge it, we couldn't get the bonnet closed. It took us ages to fix.

"It's half past eight, Kate!" the charge nurse admonished me as I rushed in, hot and flustered. "*Et pourquoi?* And why?"

I looked around in the recesses of my brain for the French word for car bonnet.

"So sorry I'm late this morning," I replied. "La capote got stuck."

The correct translation is *le capot*, which is masculine, without an *e*.

La capote (with an *e*)… is a condom.

One of my adorable colleagues, Véronique, eventually plucked up the courage to tell me that something had to be done about my speech. It was getting me into too much trouble. The hospital was thinking about kicking me out. Listening to Christophe's *argot* obviously wasn't doing the trick.

Firstly, she suggested, why didn't I take some lessons?

I signed up for ten of them at the local language school, where they assured me I'd be bilingual in a jiffy. I wrote the extortionate cheque and turned up early and eager for my first one-to-one class. Monsieur Maréchal, "*le professeur*", seemed quite pleased at the end of the hour and proceeded to give me some homework.

"I want you to sink of a *phrase*, a sentence, that uses the conditional tense, mademoiselle. For example, If I 'ad one million euros, I would buy a big 'ouse. OK? See you next Friday. *Au revoir*, Kate."

I couldn't be bothered to "sink" of another "'ouse" sentence and lazily asked Christophe, who kindly obliged me by writing something down.

The following week, the teacher asked to hear my brilliant piece of literature using "*le conditionnel*". I stood up, proudly unfolded the piece of paper and read out loud:

"*Si ma tante en avait, on l'appellerait oncle.*"

Monsieur Maréchal turned bright pink. He threw his biro at me and told me in no uncertain terms to get out: "*Tout-de- suite!*" Right away! I'd just announced that if my auntie had balls, we'd call her uncle.

Mind you, they reimbursed me. And I haven't made a mistake using the conditional tense since.

After that, my colleagues all tried to think of a different solution. It was Véronique again who came up with the idea of me applying to do a *concours*: a sort of nationwide contest for a limited number of positions in further nursing education.

"You'll never get a place," she said, putting one hand on my shoulder. "But revising in French can only improve things."

I chose anaesthesia, never imagining I'd actually end up in an operating theatre. When the results were published, no one was more surprised than me.

"You may be the first *rosbif* anaesthesia student in the history of this city!" gawped the other contestants, looking at the announcement board.

Rosbif is the French people's popular name for us Brits because, according to them, we eat roast beef *all* the time and turn pink in the sun, just like the juicy flesh of a steak. We call them "frogs", which is just as silly. I've yet to meet any French person who eats frogs on a regular basis. Snails or oysters would perhaps be more appropriate.

The national animal to represent France is actually the cockerel. This is a bird that climbs up onto a pile of *merde* very early in the morning, screeching annoyingly to anyone within a half-mile radius that he's the boss… and sod the rest of the world.

I can't actually think of a more befitting mascot to portray them.

It turned out that through winning the concours, I had signed on for two years' tough future studying at a time and location yet to be determined, at the end of which I'd be allowed to put people to sleep.

"But you do that already," said Christophe, yawning. "Every time you start talking about babies."

It had been over two years since Christophe and I had met. I'd given up a lot by leaving New York in order to stay together, and starting a family was the logical next step. I instinctively knew that Christophe would be a great dad and couldn't imagine doing it with anyone else. We skirted around the issue, not realising that our relationship was about to encounter a major test.

Christophe's company, an international fruit-trading corporation, was moving him from Paris to Antwerp, one of

Europe's largest commercial harbours. As I equated Antwerp with diamonds and Belgium with chocolate, I immediately said yes to the move, not realising that there were to be other, less digestible aspects to this new country.

The cardiology ward decided to throw a little goodbye party for me. Fabien, our Head Nurse, along with the rest of the team, clinked a toast, wished me well and said they'd miss my *bêtises,* stupid mistakes. During our farewell chat, Fabien informed me that he had bought a baby kitten for his children and decided to give it a nice English name: "Slag".

When I enquired after this unusual choice, he told me, "I 'ave a cousin in Manchester and 'ee tells me this is a cute word." Hmm... I wondered if that person was somehow related to my old nursing friend, Rob.

"Fabien," I said. "You can't call a kitten that. Do you know what slag means?" When he replied in the negative, I decided to explain.

"A slag, Fabien, is someone who has no moral values whatsoever and is capable of shagging ten different people over the course of one evening alone, in some sleazy nightclub toilets."

"Aha!" said Fabien, stroking his chin. "Then zis is an *excellent* name. It will impress all my friends. We'll keep it."

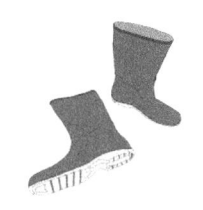

5. ANTWERP

Diamonds sparkle even under the greyest skies

The French say that Belgium is populated solely by the cerebrally challenged. I find this a bit harsh. Then again, what nation in the world doesn't have its designated scapegoat to loathe and despise? After all, the Brits bully the Irish, the Americans mock the Poles, the Greeks hate the Turks and the Japanese scorn the Chinese for being filthy and ruthless. So, if the French chose to crack jokes about the Belgians, I wasn't ready to chastise Christophe for entertaining – unjustified and misplaced perhaps – patriotic resentment against a smaller, friendly, neighbouring country.

To some degree, it appeared to be yet another national sport, like striking, tax evasion, smoking in your face and cheating on your partner; the French have probably come up with more *blagues Belges*, jokes about the Belgians than they have names for cheese.

From what I gathered, this all started with Coluche back in the '70s. He was a famous French stand-up comedian who made it big by imitating Belgians stuffing mussels and chips (the national obsession) into their babies' milk bottles. Coluche almost made it to the presidential elections in 1981; only in France could a one-man comedy show potentially run the nation for seven years, then suddenly die amid multiple conspiracy theories.

It was fair to say that there were some pre-existing conditions in place when Christophe and I decided to move into our first-storey, one-bedroom flat in Beldhoverstraat. He would have to look after the finances until I found a job, and no *way José* was I doing any cleaning, cooking or ironing.

The biggest problem is that Belgium, which is not much larger than Wales, is run by three different governments. One rules over Flanders, another deals with the French-speaking Walloon part (who, by the way, hate the Flanders lot), and both of them are controlled by a federal state. Then there's the capital Brussels, which is run separately. When you ask anybody in Belgium who's responsible for what, quite frankly, nobody has a clue. And what's worse, nobody seems to give a shit.

We soon noticed, for example, that all the streetlamps in Antwerp faced the wrong way. So, when the sun went down – rather, when the pale grey sky went dark – and the lamps were turned on, they were supposed to usefully illuminate the city's streets and pavements. Instead, tufts of grass, wasteland and walls were lit up all night. But no one seemed to think it was *their* responsibility to turn them back round the right way.

Another illustration of this daft administration was the tram doors. In the central part of the city, there is a ring road (the *rocade* pronounced *rock hard,* chortle) around which navigates a tram service. An engineer with half a brain would have placed the tram lines on the *outer* rather than the *inner* lane, thus preventing travellers from having to dodge traffic and turn into roadkill every time they tried to get on or off. But no...

The complexities of the Belgium political system were less of a concern to us, however than getting all our furniture delivered on time and in full to our new residence. We measured the collective struggle of a nation when we received a phone call from our movers asking for a Belgian *residency certificate,* needed to clear our furniture for passage, which was held up at the French border in a removal truck. This seemed like a rather insignificant red tape exercise, so I simply called the burgomaster, the town-hall office clerk, to request the magic paperwork.

"Yes, madame, it won't be a problem at all to get your *certificat de résidence*. Just give us the address, and we will send our district officer to verify that you do indeed live there."

It all sounded a bit too easy, so I risked the obvious: "Sure... um... but... we are actually staying in a hotel, precisely because our furniture, including a bed which we commonly use to sleep in, is presently stuck at the border. No *certificat de résidence*, no furniture. And without furniture, your district officer won't find us living there... on a bare floor within four empty walls."

"*D'accord,* madame, however, I *still* need to send the district officer to check that you effectively live at the address where you say you live."

Deep breath. "OK. Then how about we agree to meet the district officer at a specified hour? He would then be welcome to visit the empty flat and issue the certificate?"

"Actually, madame, no, this is not possible. The district officer decides when he will come. It's an investigation without warning, you see... to prove that you really live at the address." "Well..." I ploughed on, hopefully. "Can I just fax you a copy of the tenancy agreement?"

"No, no. The rules are the rules. Only Antwerp's district officers are allowed to issue residency certificates."

After ten minutes of this hopeless discussion, I gave in. I had already devised a secret plan: to erratically occupy the empty flat, hoping that the district officer would pop in while I was there. After a week and no sign of him, I decided to call the burgomaster's office again. With a sentiment of panic upon hearing my name, they put me through to my administrative nemesis, who solemnly confirmed the worst.

"Well, madame, let me explain... this is very unfortunate. Our District Officer, *Mijnheer* (Mister) Boris, came on Wednesday morning to the apartment, but there was nobody there! So you see, we cannot give you the certificate."

I felt like punching the wall. And the burgomaster. And Boris. This circus went on for about three weeks, after which point Christophe's company, fed up with settling hotel bills, appointed a lawyer who eventually managed to get the certificate. This cost the company about 3,000 francs. And I thought the mafia only existed in Italy! At last, though, I could move into our new home with my lovely Frenchman, no longer having to spend hours napping on a hard, cold wooden floor, waiting for a surprise visit from Boris the Belgian.

Antwerp is in the Flemish part of the country, where they speak, or rather spit, a guttural mixture of English, German and French. I could work out a few words: *stofzuiger* is a hoover; stuff sucker (ironically logical after certain A+E encounters in Brighton), *marktplaats* is marketplace, and *smakelijk* means yummy (smacked lips). The food was good, if a little unvaried, although, after a while, I couldn't even look another mussel in the face. But we never got tired of their huge range of beers and took to exploring the city's bars in the evening, intent on trying them all.

Antwerp was all but destroyed during the last war, leaving the way for tasteless constructors to build tasteless flats. A few of the original buildings still exist, and the roads are paved with old, shiny, round stones (lethal if you're in heels, by the way), giving the city an eerie, cold war, Eastern- bloc feel. A revolting, widespread child abuse case at the time served to heighten the overall unpleasantness of the place for us.

If I could give each city a colour, London would be trendy black, New York a sparkly gold, Paris a romantic, soft pink and Antwerp… grey. The sky, the streets, the rivers and the sea; different shades just seemed to merge into one. Christophe and I had permanent bronchitis due to the chilly, damp climate. We looked wistfully south towards Paris and Montpellier, trying to get away every possible weekend on the TGV to either one or the other.

I was putting all my efforts into trying to find employment. Nursing was a no-go; fluency in French and Dutch was required. The thought of trying to learn another language quickly, having not even mastered the last one, was out of the question.

Belgium's healthcare system, however, is one of the best in Europe. Mandatory insurance allows residents to access subsidised services. Belgium, like the UK, spends around 10% of their GDP on health expenditures. It is organised at regional and federal levels, funded by taxes and social contributions. The system is based on freedom of choice and equal access, as in neighbouring France. Nurses' salaries are, however, more generous (i.e. normal), averaging 63,000 pounds per year.

Searching for a career change whilst daydreaming on the TGV, I even thought about train driving for a while; you needed no formal qualifications, just half-decent eyesight. The training was free, and the pay was well above that of a nurse. To top all this, French train drivers could retire at forty-five! And they regularly found something to strike about, further enhancing their generous holiday allowance.

After much reflection, I turned to the option of teaching English and landed myself an interview at the Love English! school, located in the Stadsplein. This'll be a doddle, I told myself. After all, it's just *English*. What I speak good already, innit.

I was welcomed in the lobby by the teaching director, Mr Eurtwehoven, a very pleasant man in his thirties with smiling blue eyes. So blond he was almost albino.

"Velcome!" he said, showing me into his office on the ground floor. "Sit down, please, and take a shit."

"I *beg* your pardon?"

"Brigitte!" he yelled out to the secretary. "Bring me some

shits of paper, a pencil and a copy of ze test…"

I started to get a cold, worrying feeling in the pit of my stomach. Test?

As soon as I saw the questions, it was obvious I was going to fail; grammar was not my forte. Give examples of modal verbs. Explain the present progressive tense. Cite the grammatical difference between much and many… I couldn't answer any of them.

Looking up from the unmarked paper at Mr Eurtwehoven, we both understood it was hopeless. I'd be more capable of teaching quantum physics than English. Feeling embarrassed and deflated – I no longer felt able to run a bath… never mind a language course – I mumbled an awkward, "*Excuus*. Goodbye." I picked up my bag and put on my coat to leave.

"No, no… stay, pleeeze!" He jumped up and closed the door, looking behind him conspiratorially.

"We can, 'ow you say… come to an *arrangement*? Forget ze stupid test! *Normalement*… every-zing is OK."

It turned out that English teachers in private Antwerp language schools were a much sought-after commodity. Mainly because there were an infinite number of potential students willing to pay high prices, alongside scarce teachers who would be willing to accept a pittance.

"I give you ze job, but you 'ave to tell ze students zat you are from Oxford University, wiz a degree in literature… OK?"

Despite the obvious immorality of this offer, I shook hands on the deal. After all, this was probably the only employment opportunity I'd get. I was given an old instruction manual and told I was to start classes the next morning! Yes! Result!

"The only sing left for you to do now… is ze bonk," he said.

"*Excuse-moi?* I'm not bonking *anyone!*" I was about to call him a saucy sod and tell him to stuff his job, when I realised this was in order to organise getting paid; I had to go to the *banque*, pronounced bonk. Of course.

As I opened the door to the classroom the next day, I was shaking with fear. Ten pairs of hostile teenage eyes drilled holes into me as I sat down. I blurted out the Oxford bullshit, blushing and glancing guiltily up at the microphone on the ceiling. Monsieur *Le Directeur* listened to and recorded everything.

I introduced myself, going round the table to get to know everyone and blundered my way through the first thirty minutes session. Most of these gap-year kids were from rich families, all paying a fortune for their little treasures to obtain a fake diploma, having flunked English at normal school.

Along with my manual, I had picture cards of everyday situations that we were supposed to discuss as a group. I picked one out at random: the kitchen.

"So, everyone. What happens in the kitchen?"

"I look for a fuck in ze keetchen."

"Fork, Sebastian, *fork*…"

"Today, in ze keetchen, I whip ze balls." "We *wipe* the *bowls*, Melanie…"

"What about you, Pierre?"

"Me? I put my dick in ze dickwasher."

And so it went on. Many of my students turned out to be really quite sweet, so I tried to make the classes fun, got to know them and worked hard to improve their level of English. The methodology was simple: the students mechanically repeated what the teacher said until they got it right. It was a system for monkeys, but it worked.

Once I'd paid my bus fare to and from work, I had about twenty centimes left from my pay check each month. Not enough for even half a potato. But it was a useful pedagogic experience and just about stopped me from going stir-crazy in this depressing, grey, wet universe.

I kept the same group for just under a year, and at the end, they all got their precious, albeit useless, awards at a swanky cocktail party arranged by the school (once all the cheques had cleared) and handed out by Miss Belgium herself.

Times must have been hard, bless her.

Christophe, in the meantime, had been acting strangely. I felt like he was hiding something.

"Cherie!" he called one Friday morning. "Pack a suitcase, we are leaving for ze weekend." But instead of driving to the station to catch the train to Paris as usual, I found myself on the *autosnelwegen* heading out to Brussels International Airport. He refused to say where we were going. It wasn't until we entered the departure gate marked JFK that I understood. I threw my arms around his neck, shrieking with glee.

"Wow, this is such a *great* surprise! Woohoo! New York, here we come!" Holding Christophe's hand tightly, I could hardly keep still in my seat all the way.

Eddy and George were there to meet us at the airport. First big surprise: a baby bump was showing under her huge, pink, fake fur coat. We hugged each other so hard that I almost lost my breath. "You look amazing! I've missed you *so* much. Congratulations!" I told her.

"Aye, the wee bairn's due in January. It's greet being preggers. Ma boobs are enormous!"

We drove along I-495 West, then through the Queens-midtown tunnel, coming up out of it into the daylight to glimpse the first skyscrapers and the treetops in the park and to smell those old New York smells – it was just *so* good to be back. We entered an underground car park at 72nd Street and 2nd Avenue. Their swish apartment was on the top floor, a huge nursery in full progress. George was a legal consultant, and they were obviously doing well for themselves. Eddy had arranged a dinner party in town for us with some old hospital pals.

Christophe told them we'd meet the gang at eight after freshening up and going for a drink, just the two of us, for old times' sake. He hailed a cab and whispered the address to the driver so that I couldn't hear. I was told to keep my eyes closed. When I opened them, about thirty minutes later, we were coming up by the Hudson river, just past Chelsea market. We got out of the cab, and I recognised at once the building in front of us, even though it was the first time I'd seen it in daylight. We were back at Hogs and Heifers… the place we'd met almost three years before.

There was no sawdust on the floor now. The place had cleaned up, and there were hundreds of bras behind the bar, ours no longer visible under the great heap. Christophe ordered two glasses of champagne, and we sat down in a corner booth. He was looking restless, a little shaky. Maybe it's the jet lag, I remember thinking, he'll be OK once he's had something to eat.

He looked at me with those mischievous green eyes and said, "Do you remember the last time we were in here… we pretended to be married, yes?"

He reached into his jacket pocket and pulled out a beautiful diamond ring. "How about we do it for real?"

My joyful screams not only gave him his affirmative answer but also induced the entire clientele and staff to peer curiously over in our direction.

"We're getting married!" I yelled. "Champagne for *everyone*!" Christophe put his head in his hands. "Separate bank accounts…" I thought I heard him mumble.

I was to become Madame Lesage meaning the wise, well-behaved one. A rather erroneous name for someone who misbehaves at any opportunity, but it had a nice ring to it.

It was with heavy hearts that we boarded our United Airlines flight on Sunday (Christophe was still too scared to try and book on Virgin) back to boring Belgium, with its miserable mussels, dismal skies and forlorn-looking window prostitutes.

When we arrived home at Beldhoverstraat, there were several letters lying on the doormat. One of them had the fruit company logo on the front and looked official. Christophe opened it and read it out loud. The company was restructuring and wanted to send its young, up-and-coming managers further afield from HQ.

We would be informed of our next destination shortly.

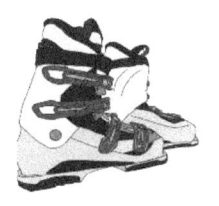

6. GRENOBLE

Girls just wanna have fun
(with anaesthesia)

We were off to Grenoble, at the foot of the Alps in South East France, and one of the main cities in the Rhône-Alpes region. Christophe's work was relocating, and we'd jumped at the chance of moving there. I immediately applied and was accepted onto Grenoble University Hospital's anaesthesia scholarship programme. We were excited about moving to the mountains; we'd had enough of flat Belgium after eleven months. We did the eight-hour long drive in our little Renault 5, stopping in Dijon on the way for a mussel-free lunch and to pick up some of their famous mustard. We took turns to drive, which was brave on Christophe's behalf as I'd not driven since passing my test in Brighton. He didn't panic, just occasionally steered us back onto the correct side of the road.

We passed a small town named Voiron, then another called Voreppe, driving into the heart of the valley. My own heart skipped a beat as the majestic snow-capped Belledonne mountain range came into view in front of a stunning pink sunset. Chamrousse ski station was signposted to the right.

Christophe haughtily told me that he had been "practically born wearing skis" (his mother's eyes must have watered, I thought), and he was eager to teach me over the coming winter.

I hoped his skiing pedagogic skills would be better than his linguistic ones. Otherwise, I was in for at least two broken legs.

The fruit company had rented us a flat in the historic town centre, furnished this time, to avoid repeating any more district officer mishaps. It was two floors up with no lift or balcony but had beautiful high ceilings and polished wooden parquet floors.

I have to admit I was a little scared about moving again, not knowing anyone or speaking the language properly. But I had my wedding to plan, and the anaesthesia course would be starting soon. That meant meeting new people, which would be a welcome blessing, even if they *were* French and would, unbeknownst to me, include plenty of sleazy Dr Neaux-type characters.

We decided to offload our belongings and head into town on foot in search of pizza. Grenoble, known as "the capital of the Alps", has a very Italian feel. Being close to the border, many Italians come over to France for work, bringing their cuisine with them. It's a large town situated on a flat plain surrounded by three mountain ranges: the Belledonne, the Vercors and the Chartreuse. Two rivers join in its middle in a Y shape: the Isère and the Drac.

Grenoble is heavily polluted, the result of being at the bottom of this *cuvette* (bowl), the extremely hot, dry summers and the many industrial plants all around, which developed at a fast rate following its holding of the winter Olympics in 1968. The local government has been run by the ecology party for many years, bravely battling the black cloud of pollution, best visible from up high.

Dotted along the *quai* (riverside) is a vast choice of pizzerias, all jostling each other for passing customers. Occasionally a bloated corpse floats down the Isère river, wearing a black shirt and a green, white and red apron, another victim of a mafia-style business dispute.

After finishing our delicious Reine and Quatre Fromages pizzas washed down with a bottle of local Mondeuse, we headed off to the famous bubble cable car and were lucky to just catch the last one up. This took us to the Bastille, over 500 metres high, where we could get a breathtaking 360° view of the city's orange roof tops and the mountains beyond.

We walked all the way back down towards the main square, *la place Grenette*, hand in hand and giggling excitedly about this new adventure that we were embarking on together. We decided to look for somewhere to go and have a nightcap. Grenoble was full of large, global companies such as Capgemini, Hewlett Packard and STMicroelectronics, who hired international people, notably Brits. These Brits, making the most of their attractive packages, lovely weather, thirty-five-hour week and seemingly unlimited holidays, could be found (at all hours of the day and night) in Grenoble's one and only Irish pub, O' Callahan's. It was packed, and everyone was swaying to Cyndi Lauper's high-pitched voice, warbling, quite rightly, about girls wanting to have fun. We squeezed in, and Christophe went to order half a Guinness and a Baileys at the bar.

"Ask if they've got any prawn cocktail crisps," I told him, ever hopeful.

I overheard English voices and turned around. A tall girl with frizzy brown hair and a beautiful smile was being chatted up by a couple of French lads.

"*Et comment tu t'appelles, toi?*" What's your name, then? One of the guys was saying, strategically leaning in towards her, one hand holding a pint, the other placed territorially against the wall above her head.

"*Moi? Je m'appelle,* Fanny!"

There was a sudden burst of shrieking laughter from across the room. The girl quickly ducked under the guy's arm to escape and went to join her friends, all of them giving each other high fives.

"That makes seven for me tonight," she said. "I win."

They must have seen me looking curiously over and beckoned for me to come over and join them. The frizzy-haired girl's name was Jodie. She introduced me to Christine, also a nurse, and Annie.

"We knew you were English when you asked your boyfriend for crisps," they explained. "They only have salt and vinegar or cheese and onion, by the way."

The game that evening, was how many times you could say the word Fanny to an unsuspecting French guy. Other favourites were Aurelie (pronounced orally) and "I'm Randy. What about you?" all of which made them chortle.

"We're always happy to meet British girls coupling with Frenchmen," said Annie. "Helps us breed them out!"

The girls had been living here for about six months. Jodie and Annie were single and working for Hewlett-Packard. Christine was married and working at one of the private clinics on a surgical ward.

"We have anaesthesia students all the time, so I'm sure we'll bump into each other," she said, writing down my number on a beer mat.

She pulled me aside.

"I have to warn you. The other nurses will look at you as if –" she searched for a comparison "– as if you've just landed from Mars. With a welly stuck on your head. And webbed feet. Just be yourself, and they'll accept you in the end." She told me that whilst on duty last Christmas day, she'd turned up for work with a pair of reindeer antlers lit up and playing *Jingle Bells* on her head. As you do. Whereas this would be completely normal, almost obligatory in UK hospitals during the festive season, the French staff thought she'd gone berserk: "A *malade mentale* (mental case), probably too much rum in ze pudding... *ces Anglaises*... tsk!" They had apparently even tried to persuade the resident doctor to refer her to the local *asile* (asylum). I was going to have to be careful.

We girls then exchanged heated views on Englishmen vs Frenchmen (out of Christophe's earshot – he was golf-bonding with Christine's husband, Tom) and on our various language bodges. We all had roughly the same lousy level of French.

Jodie's stories made me howl with laughter. It turned out she had been engaged for a short time to a guy from Grenoble and wanted to impress, or effectively suck up to his mum, by baking her something typically British. She decided on a Victoria sponge cake.

"*Madame*," she'd asked her (almost) future mother-in-law, "*Avez-vous une grosse*, do you have a large *moule?*"

She'd wanted to use the word *moule* for mould or baking tin, but it actually also means, well … fanny. And we're not talking about the name. The lady was apparently so disgusted with "zat rude Hinglish girl" that her son broke off the engagement.

Jodie then told us about another time she was on a train to Lyon. The sun streaming through the window was making her sweat. In the usual polite, English manner, she stood up to ask the whole carriage if they'd mind her lowering the window, as she was too warm.

This should have been expressed as: "*Bonjour. J'ai très chaud. Est-ce que je peux baisser la fenêtre?*" Except that she announced the ever-so-slightly different: "*Bonjour. Je suis très chaude, est-ce-que je peux baiser la fenêtre?*" Which roughly translates as "Hello everyone. I'm *really* horny… I'd like to shag the window if that's ok with you all?"

Jodie worked in an open-plan office at HP. Every evening for the past six months, she'd been popping her head up over the boarded partitions to ask loudly who was going to *ramone* her that evening? Someone eventually explained the months of stifled office snickering: what she'd actually wanted to say was the similar *ramène*, meaning 'drive home'. *Ramoner* means to shove a poker in, as one would a fireplace.

I was still chortling to myself when we got home to our new flat, happy to have met some fun, crazy people in such a short time. I had a good feeling about this place.

Before long, it was time to make my way to the anaesthetic department of the nursing school at Grenoble's CHU (*Centre Hospitalier Universitaire*). There were fifteen of us in the group. The classes were to be given every afternoon, from Monday to Friday, either by a doctor or nurse anaesthesiologist. The mornings would be spent in the various operating rooms, ICUs or with the SAMU, learning the technical stuff. One weekend out of two, plus once a fortnight during the week, we'd be *de garde* (24 hours on-call). The CHU is an enormous structure, housing every single surgical speciality, modern maternity and a world-renowned neurology department. There were even one or two Nobel Prize winners on the medical team.

Our head of teaching was a small, wiry, well-dressed man in his thirties called Frédéric. Poor Frédéric had to patiently repeat everything at least twice for the group's *rosbif*. If only I hadn't chosen German at school. He began by asking us all to talk with the person on our left for a few minutes before giving an introduction of *them* to the class.

Elliot, the guy who was on my right, was a bit slow and hadn't understood.

"What did 'ee say?" he asked me.

"We have to talk. Then, you have to introduce me," I told him.

"What?!" Elliot looked extremely offended… "On ze *desk*? In front of everybodee? But *alors*, I am a married man!" Obviously, to introduce (insert something into) someone in France was yet another *faux ami*…

The staff I met in Grenoble were dedicated, extremely competent and absolutely hilarious, and the following two years were the most fascinating, liberalising and challenging of my life. It was an emotional, academic and intellectual whirlwind.

Anaesthesia is terribly simple. Until something goes wrong. Then it's simply terrible. Anaesthetists must never, ever stop concentrating. It's an exhausting job.

As I slowly integrated into the working world of the operating room, my own grasp of *la langue de Molière* didn't fare any better than poor old Jodie's.

The drugs we administer to put the patients to sleep generally stop their breathing, so we need to hook them up to a machine called a ventilator or *respirateur* which breathes for them. If the lung alveoli are in need of a little extra filling, there's a button for what we call Positive End Expiratory Pressure, more commonly known as PEEP.

One day, we were putting a heavy smoker to sleep for a heart bypass. Ventilating his stiff, blackened lungs was proving difficult. Always on the lookout for solutions, I suggested to the doctor that a little PEEP might come in handy here. What did he think?

He turned around to face me, eyes laughing behind his mask and said, "Now, *there's* an offer I'll never refuse, Kate!" before the entire room started rolling around, clutching their tummies, tears streaming down their faces. I later learnt that *pipe*, pronounced "pip" or "peep" in French, means a blowjob.

Christophe had always told me that if ever I was stuck for a French word, to try saying the English one, then just add *er* on the end. "Nine times out of ten," he said, "it'll work... you'll see."

Once we had successfully mastered putting the breathing tube *in* (intubating), we had to learn to extubate, meaning take the breathing tube *out* again. Before doing so, one is required to suction out any secretions which may have formed in and around it using a catheter, otherwise, these can fall down into the lungs, causing infection or occlusion.

I was taking too much time extubating a patient for one

particular impatient surgeon's liking, fiddling around trying to unwrap the plastic catheter with shaky hands, all eyes on me. Students get a tough time, especially English ones.

"What the hell are you waiting for?" he yelled at me. "We 'aven't got all day!"

"I'm just going to, erm…" I stammered, trying in vain to think of the French word for the verb to suck.

So I attempted Christophe's formula of suck plus *er*.

"I'm quickly going to… *je vais vite… sucer* the patient, doctor."

"Well," he said, a broad smile suddenly forming, "at least wait for him to wake up, so he can appreciate it properly!"

My colleagues told me afterwards, whilst wiping their eyes dry, that *sucer* does effectively mean to suck… in the carnal sense of the word.

Aspirer was the word I was actually looking for. And will never again forget.

My fellow students and all the anaesthetic teams were wonderful. They nursed me, along with our patients, through two years of difficult clinical training: repeating everything over and over, helping me with the coursework, and generally showing me that our values and sense of humour were not so very different after all. Even if they *do* find Benny Hill and Mr Bean hysterically funny.

The anaesthetic doctors were a hoot and did everything to make things easier for me. Even naughty Dr Neaux turned out, in the end, to be a kind and informative mentor to whom we were all sad to say goodbye.

My favourite training area was in the *déchocage*, literally the place where you un-shock people: a two-bedded unit for uber-emergencies, most of them flown in by helicopter. I learnt so much there. Patients were generally in pretty bad shape; it was all about intubating, transfusing and scanning before heading for surgery or ICU. Relatives often waited for hours out in the adjacent corridor, hoping and praying for good news.

We'd been working on a guy in his late twenties for some time; he'd come in after colliding with a shop window, having decided to test-ride his friend's motorbike at 180km/h without a helmet *or* a license. Miraculously, he was going to be OK, apart from the numerous scars over his face, head and torso which would be left by thousands of bits of glass and gravel.

I poked my head around the door to see if any family member was waiting. At the mention of his name, a dowdy, tired-looking lady got up and came towards me expectantly, grasping her handbag tightly with both hands.

"Don't worry, madame," I told her with a relieved smile. "Your son is in a good condition, and he's going to be alright."

She gave me the filthiest of looks. I half thought she was going to spit at me.

"'*He's my 'usband!*"

On the flip side of the coin, the *déchocage* was also the location of some of the saddest tragedies that I've ever seen played out.

We got a call from one of the Dragon pilots. Dragon is the name given to France's yellow and red hospital helicopters.

"ETA three minutes. We're coming in with a two-year-old male patient, a drowning victim, weight approx. 12kgs, GCS 3. Intubated and ventilated. Oxygen saturation low. Cardiovascular status unstable." We prepared everything for his arrival in silence, any smiles wiped from our faces.

The GCS, or "Glasgow", is the coma scale we use around the world, calculated on verbal response, physical reactivity and eye-opening. The normal score is 15; 3 is the worst. It was developed, logically, in that famous Scottish town, where comas are very common on Saturday nights… after too many whiskies and a Glasgow kiss (head butt) or two.

As we put the little lad onto the table from the stretcher after counting to three, taking great care to keep his neck perfectly aligned and holding onto the intubation tube, his heart stopped beating. I immediately began paediatric cardiac massage (using the heel of only one hand instead of both, avoiding too much pressure, which can cause injury and broken ribs in children) as someone took his devastated mother aside to try and calm her down.

"I just left for five minutes to go to the shops," she was wailing. "His dad was giving him a bath, but he said the telephone rang."

The dad was pacing up and down, his face covered by his hands. Water and unsupervised children are an incredibly dangerous combination. The number of drownings and near-drownings we saw was mind-boggling.

When a child goes under in a pool, lake or bath, they simply don't make a sound.

I started sobbing, sweating from the long minutes of effort and emotion. When my colleague offered to take over, I pushed him away. We were *going* to save this kid. We had to. Nobody that young should die. After about forty-five minutes of flatline ECG, our consultant anaesthetist ordered me gently to stop.

"Go on home," he said. "There's nothing more we can do."

Looking at that lifeless, innocent face, my heart shattered into a thousand pieces. When we announced the news to his mum, she whispered his name over and over, then let out a noise I'd never heard before: guttural, almost like a wild animal.

I'll never forget it.

I took my car and drove up into the Chartreuse mountains, crying all the way.

Stopping by an empty field, I got out and ran down into the middle of it, scaring a few surprised cows.

I let out an endless scream into the valley, uncontrollably furious with myself, with the boy's dad, with a God I didn't even believe in and especially with the whole fucking unfair world.

As I often do, I pulled out my notepad and pen.

Little Angel.

I grieve for a child now who was not my own
A beautiful angel who I'd never known
Life was ahead, full of promise and joy
The games and the dreams and the smiles of a boy.

Too young and too soon to be needing a nurse
An innocent victim, no time can reverse
Oh, baby, you should have seen so many years
But you drowned. It's my turn now; I'm drowning in tears.

I tried, and I cried as I massaged in vain
The echoes of screaming; the sound of pure pain
Final gaze, final breath of your life I did share
I will never forget you, forever I'll care.

I'll remember your father, his head held in shame
I'll remember your mother repeating your name
The saddest of moments; being ordered to cease
Little angel, forgive us. You rest now, in peace...

I was lucky to be part of a group of understanding, kind professionals with whom we could all talk about the terrible stuff we saw.

There are many people working in anaesthesia who battle with depression and drug and alcohol problems, which is somewhat understandable when you're dealing with death, horror and suffering on a daily basis. Tragically, I've attended several of my colleagues' funerals over the years; all wonderful, committed, intelligent professionals... simply unable to cope.

Personally, I partied harder at weekends than I probably should have in order to forget. I cried too often, hidden in our upstairs bathroom with the tap running. I shall forever regret that nothing is done to prepare healthcare workers for the intolerable pain of losing lives, especially children.

I remember the *Nursing Times* magazine came to interview some of us Brighton students back in the 1980s. They asked what we would want to change about our training, and I remember saying that the wide availability of professional counselling would be a welcome idea, at least to help deal with all the hardship and dying around us. That was over thirty years ago, and still nothing. There should be; it's needed now more than ever.

Whereas anaesthetists are invariably fun-loving people, I found surgeons tended to be a different kettle of fish. In France, doctors are the elite of society. Surgeons consider themselves practically immortal. There was a joke at the hospital: what's the difference between a surgeon and God? God doesn't think He's a surgeon.

They have almost all attended the French elitist medical *facs,* which are extremely difficult to get into. During the first year alone, about 50% get booted out. They, therefore, have a tendency to graduate from these institutions with heads so big they have trouble getting in and out of their Porches, conveniently forgetting that they were coached, looked after and picked up off the floor the first time they fainted after seeing a drop of blood... by nurses.

Whilst watching a phimosis operation one day – a benign penis malformation – I turned to the particularly misogynistic surgeon and congratulated him on having *two* specialities.

"What are you talking about?" he said. "I am a urologist!"
"Yes," I replied. "But you're performing brain surgery at the

same time. Bravo, you."

I think he may have wanted to thump me but couldn't be bothered de-sterilising his gloves.

I also discovered that surgeons (I'll exclude female ones from this generalisation who are, thankfully, increasing in number) were absolutely certain of three things:

1. They are more important than anyone else, *especially* anaesthetists.

2. Every woman on this planet, and probably the entire solar system, wants to have sex with them.

3. The ultimate enemy of *La République Française* is the England rugby team. Surgeons, particularly Grenoble ones, are passionate about the game.

Having spent many a Saturday yelling out support to our boys at Twickenham, I am an ardent admirer of the English Roses and can belt out *Swing Low, Sweet Chariot* with the best of them, albeit totally out of tune.

Matches between our two countries became something of an issue, often quite a verbally violent one.

Someone with whom I would normally have a very civil and friendly working relationship became capable of telling me that the only good Englishman was a dead one and to bugger off back to "my island". This metamorphosis occurs during the period of the Six Nations tournament each February. By the end of March, things generally get back to normal.

Unless we win the Grand Slam, of course.

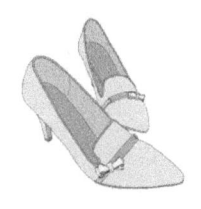

7. THE CAPE

Our Love is King

Studying one of the toughest medical specialities in a language that was not my own was nothing compared to finding my way around the complexities of the French administration system once we had decided to get married.

I got the distinct feeling that Christophe's parents had had better things in mind for their *bébé* than a crazy English nurse. He was the third of three children and the most spoiled of the brood, as is often the case.

Despite my best attempts to communicate, accept their piss-taking, wear pastel jumpers around my neck and swallow the gristly pig parts that were put on a plate in front of me on a regular basis without gagging, I didn't yet feel fully embraced into the Lesage's bosom. I began to understand the negativity towards my native country once I'd overheard a few distressing childhood memories relayed in *franglais* over family dinners.

It appears that middle-class children (my beloved included) growing up in France during the 1980s were sent to the UK during the school holidays in order to perfect their English; being able to speak English greatly improved their chances of winning a place at a superior university later on. Hosts in the UK were often working-class families in need of some extra cash. And nothing could have prepared these poor little *chéries* for the *horrific* trials and tribulations which awaited them on the other side of the Channel.

Pause for a dramatic sigh.

Their atrocious accounts of having to eat boiled meat, baked beans and jelly were equalled only by our *terrible* weather (having lived in both London and Paris, I fail to see the difference) and the general stinginess of the host families.

"You 'ave to understand, Katie, zey gave us sheet to eat!" they would tell me woefully. "Not even wine at ze table. And ze wezzer was totally crap. *Normalement* for ze 'olidays we go to Val d'Isère, Saint Trop' or Corsica… zis was torture."

"…Southampton, Leeds and Bristol are *sheet holes*. Your *yobs* were always trying to fight wiz us. And your beer is warm. *Beauk!* Yuk! Hinglish girls wear miniskirts in ze winter and are always drunk, eez dizgracefool." Etcetera. Etcetera, and accompanied by the upward palmed shrug, meaning: *now you see why I don't like you people.*

I get the jelly and spam thing; I really do. But looking round the table, everyone had attended one of the *grande écoles* (think Oxbridge) necessitating bilingual-level fluency, so I deduced that these little escapades must have served their purpose at least. Even Christophe had to admit that three months in *owful* Tunbridge Wells had helped get him into the prestigious NYU. This was worth losing a few kilos from a jelly and baked bean-based diet as well as a few teeth during pub brawls.

Most of his friends also managed to lose their virginity on these trips to England, something I would call a major success. France's younger population in those days were obsessed with a ridiculous film called *A nous, les petites Anglaises* (*Come to us, little English girls*), which portrays us as easy pickings for any horny, young Frenchman. Thus, when they arrived on our side of the water, there was only one thing on their minds involving tongues.

And it wasn't the language.

So, I had to try and think of new ways of getting accepted into the Lesage family. Kindness will only get you so far, and my humour was lost on them. It wouldn't be through cooking either, that's for sure; Gordon Ramsay, I am not. I'd already silently sacrificed ten years of secret vegetarianism. If his parents learned, on top of everything else, that I didn't like killing animals in order to eat them, I'm convinced they would have tied me up to a concrete canoe in Calais and pushed me away from the shore.

My lightbulb moment came as I was just about to click on the accept button for return airline tickets to Las Vegas. Initially, our wedding plans had been to just grab some mates and head out to the Little White Chapel for the weekend, getting an Elvis impersonator to marry us. Christophe told me that his parents were *very* disappointed not to be having the whole church shenanigans. "Too bad," I told him. "That's the way the cookie crumbles."

In French culture, it's the lady's choice. And this was no blushing Bible-bashing bride.

Christophe's stepsister Florence slouched into the drawing room, cigarette in hand, over to where I was sitting in front of the computer. Permanently bored, she was forever looking over my shoulder and asking me annoying questions in her peculiar brand of *Frenglish*.

"For ze wedding," she started, "'ow many *demoiselles d'honneur*, 'ow you say… bridesmaids, you wanna 'ave?"

My attempt at a reply in French led to another mistake. Some of us never learn. The difference between I want *trois*, three, and *toi*, you, is somewhat subtle. I needed to learn to roll my Rs more convincingly.

However, watching Florence jump up and down on the sofa in ecstatic excitement, under the false illusion that I wanted someone I barely knew by my side on the most important day of my life, *did* give me an idea. We could have the wedding in Paris and let the family organise the whole thing!

Christophe's shopaholic mother and stepsister would be overjoyed at choosing everything… all I'd have to do was try and keep it from being too tasteless. Plus, it would be closer for my friends and family to come over from the UK. The only downside for an agnostic was the fact that marrying into the Catholic Church obliged me to have some Sunday school lessons. As we wished to be married before the summer holidays, consulting the calendar, they had just over twelve weeks to save my soul.

My cunning plan came together as I had hoped. As soon as the family sniffed a religious ceremony and the freedom to organise a big, show-off party in some ostentatious château, I was in enough good books to fill the local *bibliothèque*.

The first step was trying on dresses. I was dragged around Paris's chic *7ème arrondissement* by a now very enthusiastic mother-in-law-to-be. I had an image in my mind of something extremely simple, off-white, off-the-shoulder… a little evening number from Zara. But she had other ideas. *Homecoming Prom Queen* meets *My Big Fat Gypsy Wedding* ideas. Negotiating with terrorists is generally considered a no-no. But then the FBI hasn't met Consuelo Lesage.

"Shocking!" Was her horrified reaction. "Zara? You want everybody laffin' at you?"

Coco, *all my friends call me Coco, Dahling,* imagined I'd like to resemble a taffeta and lace toilet-brush cover. After several slanging matches in front of embarrassed shop assistants, I conceded on the puffy taffeta skirt but with a sleeveless, laceless bodice. She put her chin in one hand and started tapping her cheek.

"Hmm," she said, "it *does* look nice, but eez not permitted to go into Catholic Church wiz ze bare arms! You must wear *slives*."

I checked my watch. It should still be open. We were about 300 yards from St Pierre de la Grosse Roche, the family's local church, where the ceremony was to take place. I decided to drag her over the uneven paving stones leading past the graveyard, towards the church entrance. As luck would have it, Père Brunet was in.

"Hello, Father," I greeted him. "We're here to settle a... religious dispute. The question is: Do brides have to cover their arms inside your church?"

Père Brunet peered at us both over his thick, half-moon glasses. "*Normalement*," he replied, "this is the rule. But, as you have rather pretty arms, mademoiselle... I am sure the Good Lord wouldn't mind."

Smug City 1, Paris 0.

"I must go now, it's time for Mass. Unless, of course, madame would like to confess?" This was aimed at Coco, his eyes lingering on the exquisite diamond cross falling into her ample bosom. She shook her head, mumbling something about no time, but pulled a cheque book and Mont Blanc pen out of her bag.

"So kind, madame," he said, whipping the piece of paper out of her hand before she could change her mind. "And please don't forget our *rendez-vous* next week, mademoiselle." This was directed at me. "We will be discussing the meaning of *le mariage*. I'm looking forward to it. *Au revoir, mesdames*."

As we headed back towards the car, I noticed a Parisienne clone clicking towards us down the street. Dior bag, Louboutin heels, blue fox coat and dubiously stretched skin. This one had a small dog: one of those chihuahua handbag fillers, a diamante collar clasped around its scrawny neck. Christophe always says that this type of dog is like a sample: if you like it, you can come back and buy the rest.

As they reached our car a few seconds before we did, the chihuahua cocked its skinny leg and peed all over the front wheel. Quick as a flash, Coco grabbed the lady's fur coat and proceeded to wipe the Mercedes dry with it. I dove in quickly and hid my face with both hands.

"Some people," puffed Coco, getting in next to me and

throwing the bags on the front seat, "'ave *no* manners at all."

As the driver pulled away, the shouted profanities of the damp fur coat wearer were still audible as the car turned into the next street. My future *belle mere* was a tad eccentric. But in a good way. She did make me laugh.

Coco hadn't always been surrounded by wealth and luxury, and she told me about her childhood as we drove home. Her extraordinary story is worth sharing and just goes to show that you can't always judge a book by its cover. This larger-than-life, exuberant lady was actually a heroic figure. She, along with her parents, were a shining example to people (nurses in particular) everywhere.

Born in Madrid, the youngest of three children to a beautiful haute-couture seamstress mother and prestigious tailor father, life was initially idyllic. The family were happy, hardworking and well off, and closely acquainted with the city's mayor and his family, with whom they spent a lot of time.

A few years before she was born, Coco's father, Juan, joined the Spanish Republican Army and worked his way up to become captain, a high-ranking officer in Spain. When Franco seized power in the late 1930s, their family friend, the mayor, was publicly hanged in Madrid's main square. Coco's parents and siblings were never able to remove those terrible images from their minds. Thereafter, all of the ex-regime's acquaintances were suspected of collaborating with the enemy. Coco's mother, Ariadna, and her children managed to keep a low profile to avoid arrest.

Under Franco's fascist regime, whilst her husband fought for his country, Ariadna scrounged a living by repairing soldiers' clothes. They survived the civil war but were permanently cold and hungry. Coco told me that Ariadna cried herself to sleep each night, hugging her little ones whose bones protruded through their clothes, haunted by images of genocide. She also said that pregnant Spanish women at the time who were considered, rightly or wrongly, to be communists, were forced to abort. Those who were too far gone had their babies taken away from them at birth, being falsely told that they had been stillborn. The regime didn't want children growing up as *rojos* (reds), so they were given up for adoption to "good" families. Spain was a nation cowering in terror and mistrust. Friends or even family members who disagreed with Franco were often sold out by their own to the secret police. They were then imprisoned or shot, accused of belonging to the resistance.

Captain Juan Martinez lost two-thirds of his men during the famous Madrid siege and was himself badly injured when he was shot in the knee. He was captured and imprisoned for several years, given almost nothing to eat and kept for days on end down a dark well; he regularly witnessed executions of political prisoners. Whenever Ariadna came to visit him, she first had to pay the priest a sum of money in order to be let through. The irony of Coco's recent cheque to the church was not lost on me.

He was moved from Madrid to a prison on the Portuguese border, where he discovered a strong presence of solidarity. Local fishermen smuggled in fish heads for the prisoners to eat, which saved his life, along with many others. One of his cell mates had been a dentist; this came in handy when Juan needed a rotting tooth pulling out. Juan, in turn, mended fellow prisoners' torn clothes and even stitched up their wounds.

Firstly his knee, then the whole leg, became badly infected and gangrenous from the bullet, and he was soon no longer able to stand. The guards moved him back to a military hospital outside the capital with the intention of having an amputation performed on him. Ariadna opposed the decision and begged them to let her nurse him at home. She had examined him and was sure that blood flow to the limb was still circulating; his foot had a faint pulse. In her opinion, he needed fluids, nutrients, rest and his wounds disinfecting. Juan was eventually released, broken but not defeated, into the care of his wife. Being crippled in their eyes, the army no longer considered him a threat. The family were together again, and his leg slowly healed, thanks to his wife's excellent nursing care. He began to walk again. They made ends meet as best they could, mostly by making and repairing children's school uniforms.

In 1952, however, catastrophe struck. They heard via a friend that a jealous neighbour had denounced Coco's father as a traitor, secretly siding with the communist party. The entire household was to be arrested that same night. The Guardia Civil, Franco's police force, were on their way. With just minutes to spare, they collected their few belongings and fled. Each of them were told to take just one thing: Coco chose her favourite doll, and Ariadna grabbed her sewing machine, which would turn out to be their saving grace. The men were to hike separately.

"I held on to papa so hard as I kissed his cheek goodbye. We didn't know if we'd ever see each other again."

The friend drove Juan and his brothers from Madrid to the foothills of the Pyrenees. They had managed to scrape enough together to pay an illegal ferryman, who led the men on foot through the vast, treacherous mountains to Andorra. From there, they continued on into France.

Unable to endure such a perilous journey, the girls took a night train to Perpignan. Here, they asked for political asylum and were dispatched to a refugee camp outside the town. Initially, they were given a temporary place to stay in the partially destroyed French city of Bordeaux before moving into a tiny apartment in Toulouse belonging to sympathisers.

"We had nothing to eat except a crust of *baguette* and a glass of milk each day. We shared a toilet with five other families, and all slept on one mattress. But we were finally reunited with papa – we played, we worked, we laughed. We were happy." Spanish immigrants in France at the time were considered almost as low as vermin and very much looked down upon by the locals. She told me that they were constantly mocked and bullied.

"Like the fictitious characters in Hemmingway's *For Whom the Bell Tolls*, we dreamt of a future in post-war Madrid, never imagining that we wouldn't return home," she explained. "Mama's philosophy was just to blend in, respect the rules and ignore the hateful comments. We went from being a wealthy, bourgeois Madrilenian family to being considered scum. But mama and papa were still as elegant as ever. My parents worked day and night making and repairing clothes so that we could have food on the table and get an education."

Eventually, they all learned to speak the language and obtained work permits and French citizenship. They worked and studied so hard that their family clothing and shoe business took off. They even started to export, and Coco learnt to speak three more languages.

Being in a position now to help others, they did. Refugees were still coming over in waves, fleeing the brutal war which cost 200,000 people their lives. Spanish orphans were clothed and housed, and desperate people were given jobs. She told me about one young woman who had been horribly abused at the detention camp on the Franco-Spanish border, something that happened regrettably often. Coco personally took her to a doctor, gave her a room in the family house and later made her their company manager.

Franco continued his vicious regime and was still hanging journalists until his death in 1975.

Coco met Christophe's dad at a work convention, and it was love at first sight. She was by now a divorcee, a successful businesswoman and already had a daughter, Florence. They went on to have two sons together, luckily for me. She looked me in the eye, taking one of my hands in hers. "France took us in, and it has become our home. We were so lucky to get out and come here. I truly adore this country. It has been my second chance in life. Should you ever decide to become French, remember that you will obtain rights but also duties. If called upon to respect or defend this country, we must stand together. A piece of my heart is still in Spain, but it's *La Marseillaise* that brings tears to my eyes."

The paperwork necessary for an Anglo-French wedding defies belief. First of all, you have to get hold of a *certificat de coutume*, a signed affidavit from the UK embassy in Paris. The information is given by telephone, and the average waiting time until someone answers is about five hours. If you're lucky, that is.

The *certificat de célibat*, proof that one is single, the usefulness of which is negligible, has to have a seal of approval from the Apostille of the Hague. Lord only knows why. Then you must visit a *notaire* (notary) whose preposterous fee makes you start to think twice about the whole wedding thing, in order to write your prenup agreement. Under French law, there is a choice of marrying under something called the community of property or *Séparation des Biens*. As I didn't understand a word of either, I just wrote my name as told on the piece of paper that was put in front of me. I still haven't got a clue to this day what it was that I signed.

Then, I needed to get hold of the original copies (an oxymoron if ever I saw one) of my passport, proof of address and witness details, all checked and stamped by another well-fed notary with a Seychelles suntan. The birth certificates have to be originals, including those of the bride and groom's parents. If any one of these people happens to be deceased, the computer refuses the dossier, and you are faced with a day, or maybe two, of queuing up at the aforementioned embassy to try and convince them to help. Which is about as easy as it would be convincing a nun to dress up as a leather-clad dominatrix.

If you make it thus far, the civil ceremony takes place at the local town hall, only after which can the church give its approval for the religious part. Every British document used must be translated by a designated translator into French at sixty quid a pop. Per page. Per side. And they always ask for two copies, just in case.

My theory is it's a test; if you can make it through the myriad of paperwork, avoid bankruptcy and not be deterred by this administrative nightmare, the marriage might just work.

Eventually, the time came to meet with Père Brunet and try and convince him of my being worthy enough, as a second-class Anglican, of marrying a Catholic. All I knew about them was what my Irish friend Helena had told me, "In our religion, the one who suffers the most wins." Didn't sound too tempting.

Christophe and I sat down next to each other on the opposite side of a very old desk from the good Father. I was a little nervous, the agnostic in me being very much aware that she could be easily unveiled and cast out. After promising heartily (fingers firmly crossed in my coat pockets) to bring any eventual offspring up as good Catholic children, go to Mass regularly and be a proper wife, we got down to the nitty-gritty. What was my favourite quote from the Bible? He'd like us all to say it out loud together in joyful celebration. M*erde*. I couldn't think of anything! Christophe kicked me under the table. I wish I'd listened a bit better in religious education classes at school all those years ago in Stepney. Father Brunet looked at me with one eyebrow arched and a slight smile and started tapping his fingers on the desk. He *knows* I don't know any, I realised. A clammy sweat crept across my palms.

Over on the far wall hung Jesus on the cross. I looked up at Him for inspiration and found my thoughts wandering. He had good abs, didn't he? A real six-pack. A pervert might find the whole crucifixion thing quite erotic, what with all that tying up… which made me suddenly think of The Gimp character in *Pulp Fiction*. I had an epiphany. Aha! How well the sick mind works!

"Ezekiel 25:17," I proudly announced. "The path of the righteous man is beset on all sides by the inequities of the selfish and the tyranny of evil men…" Before I could go on, he raised his hand to silence me.

"Don't think that just because I'm a priest, I'm not a Quentin Tarantino film buff, mademoiselle. OK, moving along…" he continued with a disappointed sigh, as I blushed a guilty shade of crimson.

"Next question. What is the difference between heavenly and terrestrial love?"

"Hmmm…" I drew another blank and received another kick.

"Well," he said, "let me tell you, mademoiselle. The heavenly Father will love you for all eternity. Your future husband here will love you for…" he shot a look at Christophe. "Five… maybe six minutes." The two of us cracked up as Christophe sat scowling with his arms folded. God love him, this was definitely the priest for me.

Once we had the church's seal of approval, it was time to hunt for a venue. Being in Grenoble most of the time, I had to leave this task entirely in Coco's hands, firmly stipulating that we didn't want anything too fancy or expensive as a guideline. If I'd let her have her way, we'd be dancing round the Palace of Versailles in Louis XIV wigs.

She came up trumps. I got a call from her telling me about a boat moored on the Seine, used for children's theatre shows. Very low-key, with only enough space for eighty or so people, they were willing to cut the price tag as long as we used their band for the music. I immediately agreed. After all, surprisingly, the Brand New Heavies hadn't got back to me.

I travelled up to Paris on my next day off to visit the boat and discuss the seating plan. Problem number one was putting my parents outside strangling distance of each other, and trying to avoid at least one of them going "accidentally" overboard during the course of the evening.

A certain Madame Desaulles was there to meet us on the quay. Extremely flamboyant and enthusiastic, I liked her immediately. As we crossed over the plank leading onto the boat, she turned to me and said, "I 'ope none of your party 'ave… *mal de mer*?" (sea sickness).

Being out of Coco's earshot, I replied, "Only me. I've got *mal de belle mère*!" (mother-in-law sickness). As she sniggered, I felt very proud, even if it was a bit mean and not at all true. Hurrah – my first French joke was a success!

The venue was perfect, so we booked it and put down a deposit. The rest of the weekend was spent organising hotels, flowers and bridesmaids' dresses and putting together small packets of chocolate-covered almonds called *dragées*, a traditional gift offered to each guest, placed in a small, colourful bag and tied with a ribbon.

As I travelled back on the TGV to Grenoble, I felt like we were almost ready. There was just the question of the hen and stag parties. Mine was to be a laid-back affair in London, just my favourite Moroccan restaurant with a few close friends. I had an uneasy feeling about Christophe's, though. Knowing his mates, they weren't going to let him get away lightly. I was hoping to walk down the aisle with someone who still had eyebrows.

They struck when we were least expecting it.

A few weeks before the wedding, we were finalising arrangements with the local Parisian town hall and got a call from Christophe's parents to meet them for lunch at a bistro in the *16ème*. They had reserved a table in the upstairs room and were already waiting for us, along with Christophe's brother and stepsister. We sat down and started chatting about my favourite subject: how abominably ugly all of Christophe's ex-girlfriends had been.

Tucking into my delicious sole meunière, I didn't realise we had company until it was too late. Eight masked men came bounding up the restaurant stairs and grabbed Christophe off his chair. My jaw was hanging open, half-chewed fish visible for all to see, everyone else at the table in fits of conspiratorial giggles. They stripped him almost naked, much to the other guests' amusement and forced him to put on a wetsuit, snorkel and flippers.

My fiancé was known to his buddies as *le pêcheur*, the fisherman. Less to do with his ability to catch fish than his favoured, rather revolting, joke about a fisherman's wife and her intestinal worm issues.

Over the wetsuit, they pulled on a white T-shirt depicting a smiling haddock on the front. With a wave in my direction, they carried him back down out of the restaurant and into the street, where a small group of curious onlookers had already gathered. We heard shouts and the screeching of tyres, and that was the last I was to see of him for the next forty-eight hours.

"Don't look so worried, dahling," Coco said. "Ee'll be back in one piece soon, I'm sure. This calls for one sing… *le shopping*!"

Good call. I liked that song. It had become one of my favourites.

It was on the way back home to Grenoble on Sunday that my tired, greenish-tinged fiancé filled me in on the story of the weekend's events (the bits that he could remember, anyway) in between running to the train's toilets to throw up.

The first stop had been the luxurious, famous five-star Parisian hotel: *le George V*. Christophe, by then fortified with several shots of Jack Daniels, was told to go to reception in all his scuba gear and ask for a suite with a swimming pool. He waddled up to the front desk in his flippers. The admirable clerk didn't bat an eyelid at his strange request. "I'm sorry to inform you, sir," he said. "But Monsieur Jacques Cousteau is already occupying the room. We would, therefore, cordially invite you to leave the premises."

The next stop was the fountains of the Trocadero. These are situated in a long, open basin leading towards the Eiffel tower, housing numerous fountains which continuously spurt water high into the air. Christophe was instructed to swim the length of this basin and back, something rather dangerous, not to mention highly illegal. But the brave lad was not to be deterred and accomplished the feat to applause from his friends, quite a few tourists and a couple of bemused *gendarmes* (police officers).

After drying off, he was taken across to the Eiffel tower, where he had to sell tins of "authentic" French tuna to as many unsuspecting Japanese tourists as possible. He actually made a fair bit of cash. Lastly, they drove to their favourite bar in the Place de la Bastille, where, in return for doing the washing up in his mask and tuba, he was plied with free drinks.

There, his memory fades. I can only imagine… but I prefer not to.

Back in Grenoble, it was business as usual at the hospital. I was on my SAMU (ambulance service) part of the anaesthesia internship. This basically consists of hanging around playing cards, checking that all the medicines aren't out of date for the hundredth time, cleaning out the ambulances and watching crap French daytime TV. Until *la régulation* (coordinator) rings a loud bell, indicating that you've got thirty seconds to get your arse into one of the white trucks. We were timed from that moment on. Saving patients is a race against the clock, that famous golden hour again.

The ambulance drivers' game of choice was getting students to throw up, so they floored the accelerator and exaggerated every turn. The success rate was high, as the winding roads around Grenoble were often treacherous and narrow. Student nurses and doctors were put in the back. With neither a seat nor a seatbelt, we just held grimly on to anything we could find, literally for our lives, trying to swallow down the bile rising in our throats.

Generally, patients call the emergency medical services (999 in the UK, 911 in the USA, 15 in France, 144 in Switzerland), but often it's the French *pompiers* (firemen) who turn up first on the scene to check things out, if they are geographically closer to the caller. The fire officers I met were lovely, well-trained in first aid and extremely competent. It's a good system.

In the SAMU vehicle sits an experienced driver, a specialised doctor, a nurse and the poor standing student(s). The other team members tolerated us as long as we carried the heavy stuff and acted as human drip stands. I loved getting out and about. Seeing patients in their homes made a nice change from on operating room tables. Our job was to assess the situation, treat the emergency and decide whether or not to bring the patient back to the hospital.

Chest pain is the trickiest one. It can signify life-threatening conditions such as myocardial infarction, aortic aneurysm, infection of the heart or lungs, pneumothorax or pulmonary embolism. Often, there are serious gastrointestinal causes, such as gallstones, a bleeding gastric ulcer or pancreatitis.

Some of the time, though, it's either psychological or a bit of trapped wind, departing miraculously after the patient has had a good burp or fart. This frustration can occasionally cause a nonchalant approach to chest pain by SAMU medical personnel, which might explain the following situation.

We got a call from *la régulation* at around three o'clock one late spring afternoon. A forty-year-old female presented with quick-onset chest pain radiating down the left arm. The address was one of the local ski stations – profession: chalet cleaner. No past medical history, no medication except Xanax for anxiety and no risk factors apart from smoking about ten cigarettes a day.

Most of the SAMU staff I met were extraordinarily devoted and talented. But today, the young on-call locum emergency doctor was an arrogant, egocentric gung-ho type. In France, they call these guys *cowboys*. He was in the middle of an episode of his favourite French television series, *Fort Boyard*, and had no wish to be disturbed.

"*Non! Mais… putain!*" he complained, using the worst expletive in the French language – a word for prostitute. I have no idea why they should be thus degraded; they're just trying to do a job like everyone else.

"Another bloody hysterical young woman, wasting our time and resources. It's in her head, you mark my words."

"Or maybe it *is* cardiac in origin," I said, reaching for the rolled-up pack of emergency meds, oxygen and mini defibrillator. "Anyway, we're obliged to check it out. Come on."

"You just leave that right there," he instructed me, pointing at the material. "I *forbid* you to take it, Kate. A complete waste of time."

As a student anaesthetic nurse, I had to obey the doctor's orders unless they were clearly illegal, so my conscience was presented with a moral dilemma. Either we arrive at the scene without the necessary gear, or I get kicked off my internship in disgrace for disobedience.

As it was, he solved the problem for me. "We'll take the helicopter. That way, I'll be back in time to see the end of my show."

Talk about wasting resources, I thought.

This was a big thing for me: my first time in a helicopter. I have to admit it was very exciting. I'd been waiting two months for the experience. At any time of year, it gets extremely cold once you're up at a certain altitude. I was therefore lent a huge, black, leather poncho with SAMU 38 written on the back in big, white letters. Plenty of room to hide whatever I wanted underneath.

"I 'ope you've got your furry knickers on, *l'anglaise*," the pilot shouted to me. "It's freezing up zerre!"

Distracted with excitement, I committed the *erreur de débutante* – beginner's error – and walked around the back of the whirring helicopter to climb in. They told me afterwards I could have been decapitated on the spot.

We flew over the valley and headed up into the Alps. It was a glorious day, and the visibility was great. It was exhilarating. We had headsets on in order to communicate with the pilot.

"Where are we going?" I asked him, looking out of the window onto snow-topped trees, my teeth chattering.

"Not sure yet," he replied. "Haven't got ze *exact* address. I sink it is at *Pipay* or *Prapoutel*." These are two of the ski stations in the Grenoble area, I later found out. But what with his accent and the radio interference, I understood that we were headed towards a destination known as *Pipayorprapoutel*.

We landed in front of a large chalet, attracting a lot of attention and spraying snow in all directions. As we entered the lobby, a group of people were huddling around a middle-aged lady, sitting on the floor, breathless and clutching her chest. As I knelt down next to her, she fell backwards, her eyes rolling upwards at the same time. She was no longer breathing, and when I checked for a carotid pulse, there was none.

"Oh, *mon Dieu!*" shouted the doctor. "She's in cardiac arrest! *Les carottes sont cuites… les carottes sont cuites!*" He started to panic, losing the plot completely. The carrots are cooked? What on earth?! Someone needed to take control of the situation.

"Well," I replied, taking the defibrillator out from underneath my coat, "we might be needing *this*, then, eh?"

My colleague was in such a state of catatonic surprise that I decided to defibrillate the patient myself. The monitor showed lethal ventricular fibrillation. Making sure that no one was touching her and having put gel on the palettes to avoid skin burns, I pressed the button and zapped 200 joules towards her heart.

Nowadays, there are simple-to-use automated external machines in many public places, but at the time, all we had were manual ones.

Defibrillating a heart is like (gently) slapping a naughty child's bottom, so they stop misbehaving and start acting normally again. The arrhythmia, most frequently ventricular fibrillation or ventricular tachycardia, is stopped by the electric current, and the heart's natural pacemaker re-establishes a normal rhythm. At least, that's the idea. This time, happily, it was successful.

The quicker the heart gets shocked, the better the outcome, and luckily we were witnesses to this particular cardiac arrest. If a defibrillator is not immediately available, start rapid chest compressions, having first called for help.

Shocking *asystole* or "flatline" doesn't work, as there's no arrhythmia to control, unlike what you may see in the movies. My medical colleague had by now snapped out of his own state of shock. We quickly put in two large IV cannulas and intubated the lady before carefully putting her onto a stretcher and hoisting it into the helicopter.

She was stable all the way back to the hospital, where the cardiac surgical team took over and whisked her straight down to theatre. She underwent emergency bypass surgery: basically plumbing the heart's blocked arteries using veins, harvested from elsewhere in the body, to go around the bunged-up bits and restore blood flow to the *myocardium*, or heart muscle. The good news was that she was fine, made a full recovery and even decided to quit smoking.

The young doc never mentioned a word to me about what had happened.

I've worked with hundreds and hundreds of doctors over the years, most of whom were humane, compassionate and incredibly knowledgeable. But the helicopter episode always reminds me of three things: listen to the patient, teamwork is vital, and *everyone* makes mistakes.

Exhausted by all these dramatic events, I plopped myself down on a chair in the anaesthesia staff lounge and helped myself to a piece of chocolate black forest *gâteau* that some kindly soul had brought in to share.

Dr Neaux happened to be reading the paper.

"So," he said, looking at me over the pages. "I hear you took an eventful trip in Dragon. Where did you go?"

Hmmm… where was it again? Ah yes. "*Je crois*, I believe… we visited… Pip… otel?"

Too late, I'd said it. Blowjob hotel. Oh, *putain merde*.

"Aha!" he exclaimed, getting up to leave. "Well, Kate, I hope you booked me a room there for at *least* a month."

The second time I went up in Dragon, I was in for another unforgettable experience.

We were called to help the mountain rescue team, but this time not to find the usual off-piste skier seeking perfect white powder, but a fifty-eight-year-old woman who had taken an overdose of barbiturates, stripped stark naked and headed off to the local hills in the middle of the night. As she had not been spotted since, there was fear she'd been caught in an avalanche. Avalanches are a frequent occurrence in the mountains, especially in late winter and early spring. Victims' chances of survival, I was taught, depend, amongst other things, on whether or not we find snow in their mouths.

If this is the case, the odds are slim, as they would most likely be suffering, or even have died, from hypoxia (a lack of oxygen). However, if their airway is free, the patient may just have severe hypothermia and still be in with a chance. Hypothermia can be reversed by several warming methods, notably extracorporeal circulation, where the body's entire blood volume is passed through an external warming machine.

We had to find and extract the woman's body using long sticks and dogs.

"Don't forget, if you ever ski off-piste," the doctor beside me said, "always have something smelly in your pocket... like an old sausage. That way, the dogs will find you more quickly."

Since hearing that, Christophe and I always pop into the butchers for a couple of stinky *saucissons* on our way up to the slopes.

My stick hit something hard.

"*J'ai trouvé quelque chose!*" I've found something, I shouted. It was our lady. And, even better, her mouth was snow-free.

We dragged the woman's bloated, ice-blue body out of the snow and quickly whisked her into the helicopter, immediately covering her with a shiny, gold emergency blanket. Being a lady of rather large proportions, the pilot told us that someone would have to find other means of transportation home; Dragon can only hold a certain weight. All eyes fell on me; the least important person there. It took me three hours to clamber back down the mountain and find a bus all the way to Grenoble. Bastards.

I went to visit the patient upon my return. She'd been bled out, warmed up and saved. The mixture of barbiturates and freezing cold had completely preserved her brain and other vital organs. Historically, it was one of the few totally successful recoveries from such a low temperature for many years. Articles of her rescue were to be written in the most prestigious medical journals… the hospital emergency department was in ecstasy.

She was sitting up in bed, flicking through *Voici* – the French equivalent of *Hello* magazine.

"Bonjour, madame," I introduced myself, explaining the part I'd had to play in her rescue. "I hope you're feeling warm, well and making a good recovery?"

"I don't know why you bothered," she told me stonily. "I wanted to end it all, and you prevented me. As soon as I'm out of here, I'll have another try. Bloody do-gooder."

I went home that evening and poured myself an extra-large G and T.

Luckily, I didn't have too much time to dwell on all this drama, what with the wedding approaching. There was still lots to do. I was relieved and happy beyond words that most of our closest, beloved friends and family could make it. Work had agreed to give me two weeks off, so the honeymoon had to be somewhere not too far away, minimising potential jetlag. A dear friend of the family had contacts at a luxury glamping site in the Kruger National Park and graciously offered to pay for five nights there as a wedding present. Neither of us had ever been to South Africa.

We booked air tickets to Cape Town and organised the safari, a tour around the vineyards of Stellenbosch and a trip down the Cape Flower Route.

Finally, the big day arrived.

Leaving Christophe's parents' apartment, I tripped across the stony streets of Paris's *7ème arrondissement* dressed in cream taffeta to St. Pierre's, arm in arm with my dad, followed closely by Jo, Julia, Eddy and Christophe's stepsister Florence, all holding the train.

Père Brunet was on the steps to meet us. "Nice arms!" he said with a wink.

Entering the magnificent gothic building, my eyes immediately fell on Christophe's sweet little nervous face at the altar turned towards me. During the ceremony, I didn't understand a single word, probably due to stress, despite having revised my lines every night. Christophe just pinched me, as arranged, whenever I had to say, "*Oui.*"

Coco had obviously had a hand in Christophe's wedding suit; he looked like he'd just stepped out of a Dickens novel.

We both found it difficult to stay serious during the long ceremony, having the odd outburst of nervous giggles which drew dagger looks and the sign of the cross from my new mother-in-law. Once we'd exchanged rings, sang the last hymn and heard the final reading, we exited the church as *mari* and *femme*. We descended the steps to the sound of chiming church bells, cheers and whistles from our nearest and dearest all around us, under a shower of red rose petals and rice. I was gagging for a glass of champagne. Luckily one of my old East End mates had opened a bottle. He handed me a flute full to the brim.

"Quick Kate," he whispered. "Get that down your Gregory Peck (neck)!"

This gave me the necessary Dutch courage to face the camera: I hate having my photo taken. Putting on a frozen smile on the steps of the church, I posed with Christophe for what seemed like an eternity in order to fill albums with traditional marriage images, enough material with which to bore generations of Lesages for hours on end, at future family gatherings.

As we headed back down the church steps together, I noticed three old-fashioned buses parked at the side of the road by the gates. I had understood that we were all taking taxis to the boat, but Coco had come up with another fabulous surprise. The Paris public transport department had kept hold of a few of these 1920s treasures, and she had somehow managed to get her manicured hands on them for the day. They were a beautiful dark green colour, with a cream top and matching leather seats.

The first-class area had a roof over it, whilst the people in second-class had to stand at the back in the open air, with nothing but a pole to hang on to, just like those London buses back in the not-so-distant past. I headed for the rear, climbing, unladylike and barefoot, onto the first bus, bridesmaids in tow and still clutching my champagne glass. Twirling around the pole, it was a bit like being at Save the Robots club in New York. All the other guests scrambled on, and as the convoy headed off, the loud clanging sound of empty tin cans on the cobbles followed us.

The buses couldn't do more than about 15mph, so we were able to savour the sights of Paris as well as the look on everyone's faces on the streets. Coco had thought of everything! Plates of *saucisson* and paper cups full of Beaujolais were passed around as we drove by Les Invalides, admired the Eiffel Tower and Champ de Mars, where Christophe had bravely swum not long before, then passed over the Seine via the Pont d'Alma towards Place de la Concorde. Finally, the buses parked in front of the Louvre museum, its stone glowing pink in the sunset across the road from where the theatre boat was moored. We all disembarked.

A young lady in her twenties called Charlotte welcomed us, taking everyone's coats and presents to be held in the boat's cloakroom. Then, one by one, we were escorted across the gangplank by Madame Desaulles. There was a jazz band gently playing as a backdrop for cocktails and chatting before we sat down for the meal (strictly according to Coco's seating plan, of course) down in the galley. As dessert was being served, there was the clinking of spoon upon crystal to announce the best man's speech. Christophe's brother stood up.

"Uh oh," I said to myself, taking a large swig of Calvados brandy. "Here we go. At least his accent is pretty good. My lot might even understand."

Guillaume cleared his throat.

"When my brother announced he was marrying an English girl," he started, "the whole family was obviously very shocked."

Ripples of nervous laughter from the French. Tutting from the Brits.

"Then, he told us that she was a nurse. As Christophe faints at the sight of a needle, the slightest drop of blood or any other bodily fluids for that matter… we did not understand. He will never, for example, change a nappy. *That's* for sure."

Faint chuckling at the back. Come on, Guillaume, you can do better than that.

"But when we heard she was a blonde… well, it defied belief!"

This induced much banging of hands on tables and slapping of Christophe's back by his mates. He'd always been obsessed with dark Spanish types before me. His ideal woman was Penelope Cruz. Who, sadly, I do not resemble at all.

"So, without further ado, as my brother has now settled down and is taken, I must ask all of the brunettes who are still in possession of a key to his house to please return it right now."

A long line of brown-haired female guests formed in front of Guillaume, each one handing him a large key. Someone's eighty-five-year-old grandmother even played the game (wearing a curly afro wig). As did my mate Helena's six-year-old, dark-haired daughter. Luckily, everyone was drunk enough to find that (in) appropriately amusing.

We danced to our song, Sade's *Your Love is King*, before everyone, French and English alike hit the bar and dance floor with a vengeance. We rocked that old boat till well after midnight, and, luckily, nobody required fishing out of the water. Nor did anyone have *mal de mer*, for that matter.

Upon leaving, however, we found out that Charlotte had scarpered with all the coats and wedding presents. She and they have never been traced.

Apart from that little mishap, we had the best day ever.

Christophe's parents had spoiled us rotten. I will forever be so glad and so grateful for those memories… and that we didn't just pop over to Vegas.

We flew off to Cape Town the next morning. The wildlife, ocean, plants and food were like nothing I'd ever tasted, seen, smelt or experienced before. We ate the most exquisite fish, meat and fruit and drank the most glorious local wines; we watched majestic humpback whales breach from our hotel balcony. We encountered lions, giraffes and hyenas crossing the dusty tracks in the Savannah sunrise in front of our jeep. We got charged by Mad Martha: a well-known psychotic elephant in the bush who has been responsible for many a tourist peeing their pants, and we spotted Jacques Cousteau's boat, the *Calypso*, off the shores of Table Mountain (the research team were apparently going out to cage-dive amongst great white sharks). "It's a shame, his room at the George V must be free now," muttered my silly new husband as he kissed me.

The weather was perfect, the people wonderfully friendly, and the scenery exquisite. The week went by far too quickly. All too soon, it was time to get back to Grenoble. And back to nursing.

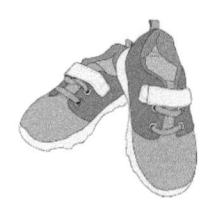

8. FROM TWO TO THREE

A baby, stitch-ups and driving fiascos

South Africa was stunning, adventurous and fertile. When we got back, I was already pregnant. A result of wedding stress relief, as Christophe put it romantically.

Luckily, my anaesthesia studies were going to be finished before the predicted delivery date. This meant not having to redo my second year, so long as I didn't screw up the final exam, of course.

At the hospital, nothing much had changed. I informed everybody of my condition because we were regularly exposed to X-rays and anaesthetic gases, which can be dangerous to a foetus. There had also been a recent intake of *cowboy* surgical interns, which would stretch my patience. I started my final gastrointestinal internship alongside one of the crazier ones. He was clever and talented but had a particularly twisted mind.

He was washing his hands one morning at the surgical sink as I went up to discuss his next patient's anaesthetic protocol. The poor woman had presented with a painful perianal fistula. This is generally due to infection and results in a small tunnel being formed from the bowel to the skin, somewhere around the anal area. She was asking for it to be done as an ambulatory procedure; where the patient doesn't spend the night in the hospital. But her diabetes was out of whack, and I thought it might be better for her to stay over, enabling us to control her blood sugar properly with sliding-scale insulin, at least until the next day. Not being my decision to make, what was his opinion?

"What eez my opinion?" he said, scrubbing even harder as he looked at himself admiringly in the mirror. "*Putain!* Imagine! FOUR holes…"

I chucked the dossier in the direction of his head, turned on my crocs and stormed out to report him, feeling nauseous.

Nausea *really* kicked in after the second month. The pregnant body changes in such strange ways, particularly its sense of smell. If someone was burning toast two miles away, I knew about it. And so did our unfortunate toilet.

What with stressful exams looming and hormonal changes, tempers at home were flying. The honeymoon period hadn't wound down gently, so much as collided headlong into a brick wall.

When I got really pissed off, I'd use the old "I don't know why I married *you!*" routine. Christophe would just wander over to the window, pull the curtains aside and mutter, "Well, I don't see a queue out there…"

In order to get out of the house and away from the old *trouble and strife* – ha! He got it now – Christophe had taken up hunting, as he called it, for mushrooms in the surrounding mountain forests, and he'd skip off early in the morning on weekends, wicker basket in hand.

One day he asked me sweetly to come with him, saying it would be good for us to "share my new passion and spend quality time together." What he really wanted me for, of course, was to smell out a truffle or two for him with my new super-nose. He actually asked me to get down on all fours in the mud and sniff. We may have met in a bar called Hogs and Heifers, but I didn't exactly find being taken for a squealing, hairy pig very flattering.

The French are phenomenally weird when it comes to mushrooms. A good basketful of *cèpes* or *morilles* is worth a fortune, and where they grow is guarded with great secrecy by the chosen few. Christophe always says he'd rather give away his bank account details than the whereabouts of one of his *morille* spots.

I was talking about this to one of my post-operative patients in recovery, who seemed to have been struck down with the same mushroom affliction.

"You know," he told me, "it's a very serious subject in this country. The information is handed down over generations, from grandparent to grandchild. You want my credit card's secret code? OK. Keys to my Porsche? No problem. But, tell you where my mushrooms grow? No way!" I guess there are some things I'll *never* understand about these people. I spent one memorable on-call weekend looking after an emergency liver transplant patient – he'd eaten a dodgy one – that put me off fungi foraging forever. Never, ever eat a mushroom that you're unsure about.

I managed to validate my internships and pass my final exams, despite all the hiccups on the way. On one paper, which was supposed to be anonymous, the cheeky examiner had written: *I recognise this accent. Hello Kate!* I guess we must write how we speak.

One of the exam questions depicted the scenario of a woman, post caesarean, who was bleeding internally: pain, pallor, heavy and constant vaginal haemorrhaging, blood pressure dropping, heartbeat rising, nausea and so on. The question asked, *"En quatre mots* (in four words), what needs to be done?"

Shit, I thought, only four flipping words? What this woman needs is: monitoring, reassurance, to be examined by a midwife and obstetrician, check that two wide-bore IVs are in place, labs and blood cross-matching done, uterine massage, O negative transfusion, IV frozen plasma, oxytocin, an oxygen mask and vasoconstrictors. Just for starters. But what will probably save her life is being opened up again to identify and clamp the source of bleeding. So, I wrote, "Back. To. Theatre. Quick." Four words, as demanded.

I didn't do very well on that question and asked the examiner why. It turns out that *en quatre mots* is just a French saying and not to be taken literally. I tried to argue that it wasn't fair; exam questions should be internationally clear, and a re-evaluation was in order! This was a scandal!

I was told, in no uncertain terms, "*Dans tes rêves et va te promener.*" Dream on and shove off.

Becoming a qualified anaesthetic nurse was the greatest achievement of my professional life. I was over the moon. I love so much about it: the autonomy, the teamwork, the simple, algorithmic logic of it all and the magic of being able to take someone's pain or worry away just with the simple push of a syringe.

On the subject of pain and pushing, my pregnancy was advancing well. I attended regular antenatal classes, learning how to inhale and exhale at all the right moments. The sickness had passed, and I could feel little elbows and knees digging and poking around inside me, reassuring signs of a feisty baby.

Christophe hadn't taken the pregnancy news too well at the beginning. It had been the classic story of being too drunk to go and fetch the condoms from the bathroom cabinet. Neither of us was expecting to expect quite this soon. I was secretly thrilled at the idea of a little baby and becoming a real family. My mother had always told me I'd be utterly crap at parenting, and I was determined to prove her wrong. Whilst I'd peed on the test stick almost nine months previously, Christophe had paced around the living room, necking neat Scotch. Seeing the little red line appear was possibly his most traumatic life event. He went deathly pale and started to hyperventilate; I had to lay him down on the sofa and give him a paper bag to breathe into. Top tip; it gets your carbon dioxide back up and may stop you from passing out.

So, hardly the joyful, blissful moment that I'd dreamed of – no giddy sweeping hugs, romantic background music and "put your feet up, Cherie, I'll make dinner" for me. About as far from those as you can get, in fact. But as the months went by, he seemed to warm to the idea. And as the time drew near, he even painted the baby's room pale blue (we knew it was a boy, and he insisted on choosing the name as well as the wall colour). I think he was even more excited by the end of the pregnancy than I was.

The final days are the worst. So I did what many bloated, fed-up, impatient future mums do: I ate an extra spicy chicken vindaloo. It did the trick. Within a few hours, the contractions had started. I excitedly called Julia, my first friend to have had kids, to ask her about childbirth: What should I expect? What did it feel like?

"Shitting out a rugby ball covered in broken glass" was her answer. Without any hesitation.

It was, therefore, with much trepidation that I packed a small suitcase with the list of things I'd been given and instructed Christophe to drive us slowly to the hospital. The local taxi company had flatly refused to pick us up, apparently more scared of a pregnant woman's waters breaking over their seats than some drunk ready to empty his guts and/or bowels at 3 a.m. on a Sunday morning. I made a mental note to sue once all this baby business was over.

The contractions were getting increasingly painful and frequent by the time we arrived. I was put in a bed, hooked up to a load of drips and monitors, and prodded and poked like a chicken being prepared for roasting. Everyone looked very serious.

The "Can you see if my lost Rolex is in there, please?" from Christophe didn't get any laughs.

Five centimetres was the midwife's verdict. Only *five*, I thought. Christ! Just halfway. I'll never make it. My midwife was actually a man, and I wondered what they called themselves – midhusbands? He was very kind. A lot of the ones I'd met professionally could be rather creepy. Did I want an epidural? All that talk of a natural birth plan, using hypnosis, yoga and massage went down the toilet as those evil contractions really got going. Yes, I wanted a sodding epidural *and* as much morphine as they could possibly pump into me.

The choice in France is pretty open when it comes to childbirth. If I'd wanted a caesarean section on a particular date, I would have probably got it, as long as I was in a private hospital and my doctor wasn't off playing golf in St Andrews that weekend. In France, women are also eligible for seven free health checks during pregnancy. They stay on average for four days in hospital, and everything is 100% reimbursed. I experienced excellent food: lots of creamy mash potato, beer (good for producing milk, they told me: bring it on!) and even a cheese course. I received my normal salary for sixteen weeks, the recommended necessary recuperation time determined by the WHO. Christophe was allowed eleven days of paid paternity leave. If we'd had a multiple birth or adopted, it would have been a lot more.

Things were really starting to move down below. I could see in my midwife/husband's face that it was lights, camera, action time. I was also starting to regret the vindaloo, although at least my special moment was impregnated with nostalgic smells from my childhood (our Indian neighbours, to be precise). "Get him the fuck out of here!" I yelled, legs akimbo in stirrups, when some bedraggled, unkempt person popped his head round the door. "I don't want some goat herder watching me give birth!"

"This is Dr Crochet, and he's a *remplaçant*," I was told.

"Your usual gynaecologist has a weekend in Scotland which he couldn't cancel, I'm afraid."

Despite his appearance, the good doctor did his job. Our *enfant cordiale*, Alexandre, came into the world at 10.28 a.m., bald as an egg and screaming his little head off. But we both immediately fell totally in love with this new person. He had two beautiful blue eyes, a button nose, and ten fingers and toes, which we counted with a sigh of relief… he was just perfect.

My very happy but slightly wobbly husband went straight out to call everyone and buy me some flowers whilst another doctor stitched me back up, surrounded by a gaggle of red-faced interns who had gathered round to watch. Talk about adding serious insult to injury.

"Unless, of course, you mind, madame?"

"Oh no!" I attempted a strained smile through gritted teeth. "Everyone's got to learn, haven't they?" Of course, I bloody well minded. My privates weren't usually open to the public.

Being left alone at last a little while afterwards, I took hold of my Evian mist water vaporiser, sat on the edge of the bed, opened my legs and prepared to spray in order to ease the stinging. Just at that moment, the door flung open, revealing Christophe clutching a bunch of wilting daffodils.

"What on earth are you doing, Kate?" he exclaimed, looking down. "Killing flies?"

I laughed so hard that they had to stitch me up again.

It's well known that the French are sex mad, but I had no idea just *how* much until the person charged with discussing post-natal contraception paid me a visit on my third day in hospital. Had I thought about going back on the pill, or would I prefer having a *sterilet* (coil) put in?

"It is a myth that breastfeeding stops you from getting pregnant, you know… one can't be too careful." Wink, wink.

"*Attendez*. Hang on a minute," I said. "My nether region has just been sliced in two. If my husband comes anywhere near me at the moment, I'll throw darts at his balls."

Actually, Christophe informed me, a large number of French women conceive again rapidly after giving birth. His own brother, Guillaume, is exactly ten months older than him. Poor Coco, the very idea made my toes curl inwards.

Apparently, it's the sort of thing a *good* wife does: making sure her frustrated husband isn't tempted to run off with his secretary. It wouldn't be his fault, either, what with her being so fat, tired and unattractive after having a baby. Not that many of them *do* get fat; putting on more than a few pounds during pregnancy is frowned upon by many French girls. As if having a human being (or two) growing inside of you isn't a good enough excuse to lose your perfect *silhouette* for a little while!

Breastfeeding is another contentious subject in France. Yes, it might be good for bonding and giving the kid its antibodies, but we can't have our boobs sagging, can we? Monsieur would not be happy.

But by far the most bizarre and embarrassing post-birth (se) x-factor is the *rééducation perinée*. Indeed, the honourable and beneficial idea behind this rather intimate physiotherapy is that it helps the pelvic floor muscles regain their pre-baby strength, thereby reducing the risk of wetting oneself when coughing, laughing or trampolining. After childbirth, it's as if your vagina *was* your closest friend, and now she's not talking to you anymore.

But let's face the truth. The primary goal is to tighten up your mangled bits and pieces in order to get back on track under the sheets. When I left the maternity ward, I was given a *rendezvous* a few weeks later with a physiotherapist specialising in the perineum. It's practised widely in France and pretty much mandatory after birth.

I turned up for the appointment, and a tall, stoic lady with her hair up in a bun asked me to take my clothes off, change into a paper gown tied up at the back and lie down on an examination table. She then put on a pair of plastic gloves and unceremoniously stuck two fingers up inside me, asking me to contract. A little surprised, I contracted as hard as I could, gritting my teeth and clenching my buttocks.

"You can start to contract now, madame… whenever you're ready."

Chuffing hell.

The worst thing is that from the pram across the room, your baby is looking straight at you throughout. Although he *is* the guilty party, it just somehow doesn't seem right. Hopefully, they don't remember at that age. If they do, we'll be spending a fortune in therapy for him later on in life.

As I was evidently not contracting at an Olympic level, she went to fetch something ominously called *le Probe*. She came back holding what could only be described as an enormous metal buzzing phallus.

"Don't worry," the physio told me. "It's all reimbursed by the state."

That was the least of my worries. No way on earth would I survive the ensuing psychological and physical trauma. I grabbed my bag and the pram and got the hell out of there fast, still wearing my gown and leaving little droplets of pee behind me, like the *Hansel and Gretel* tale with a twist.

It has to be said that perineal exercise classes are an excellent example of medicine being geared towards preventative health. One out of ten women suffer from incontinence after childbirth, and one in three have some stress leakage. I do therefore believe it *is* a good idea and even found the courage to go back to the physio after my daughter was born. Now that I'd seen what could only be described as Robocop's penis, at least I was prepared to handle the situation… by closing my eyes and thinking of England.

Organising childcare in France brings you into a whole new level of French administrative stress. If you're hoping for a place at a communal *crèche* for your little one in France, you may have the slimmest of chances if you apply before conception. Your great-grandfather's conception, that is. Places are scarcer than a virgin in one of Antwerp's seedy hotel windows.

Despite grovelling letters to, and sickly smiles at, the people who work in the *Mairie*, there was no room at the inn for little Alex. In this case, Plan B is *une assistante maternelle*, often referred to as a *nounou*. These are women, more often than not, who look after a number of children in their own homes, like a childminder in the UK.

Being a much more expensive option, this is not ideal. But for a nurse, it offers far more flexibility; *nounous* don't mind us turning up as early as 6.30 a.m. for drop off and are very understanding when we come to collect our little treasures, utterly exhausted at 7 p.m. or even later. *Crèches* generally close at 6 p.m. on the dot.

Nounous will also often take your kid off your hands if it's (a little) sick. The slightest hint of a snotty nose or temperature raised above 37.1° detected at a *crèche* invokes a panicked phone call ordering parents to fly in immediately and exfiltrate their dangerously contaminating, bacteria/virus-ridden child, which is not possible when mummy is in the middle of an open heart operation…

We interviewed several women, noticing they all gave themselves pseudonyms like Nanou, Mima and Tattie. This was supposed to make them sound maternal and cuddly, but I found the whole image unsettling, especially with their spooky old houses, complete with flapping shutters, dark cellars and creaking stairs.

Then we discovered normal-named Céline; she swept Alex

up in her arms and declared he was the *"plus beau garçon du monde"* – the most handsome boy in the world: she certainly knew how to talk to me. Her house was clean and relatively modern compared to the others. The large garden was full of toys and contented, rosy-cheeked children ran around it surrounded by colourful geraniums, rhododendrons and hortensias. There was a mouth-watering smell of creamy chicken and mushroom stew wafting out of the open patio windows. It was a warm, homely place. We hired her immediately before someone else got there first. I needed to have the reassurance that I could leave Alex happy and safe when I returned to my job. Not all healthcare workers have this luxury.

Now that I was officially qualified to put people to sleep, things were getting a tad scary in the big, wide world. We were professional anaesthetists accountable for our actions. Being totally free to prescribe and administer just about whatever I esteemed justifiable was quite a responsibility. Often, the doctors weren't present or were occupied elsewhere. Once the patient was intubated, they basically buggered off and left us to it. When we weren't sure, we beeped them. But if they were busy, we simply had to manage.

I was neither the most brilliant student nor the world's greatest nurse, and sometimes I got it wrong. Though luckily, never with dire consequences. The language didn't help. I remember speaking to an anaesthetist responsible for the operating room I was working in one day, who'd gone off to visit a patient in recovery. Despite deep anaesthesia, my patient's blood pressure was too high at 190/100. The risk, in this case, is bleeding or even a stroke. I'd tried a couple of medicines without result. So I called him up. He told me, over a rather bad telephone line, to give Loxen, a potent vasodilator.

What I *heard* was, "Give *deux* (two) milligrams." In fact, he'd told me to give a "*demi*" (half) a milligram.

I didn't have to worry about high-blood pressure after that. It came crashing down faster than the lift in *Die Hard* to about 80/40… I shoved his legs up in the air and lowered the head of the bed to get the blood running in the general direction of the brain before opening his IV at full speed in order to fill him up, like a bath.

When something like this happens, I turn bright red, my heart starts thumping, and my mouth becomes drier than a camel rider's old flip-flop. I could have done with a good dose of Loxen myself at that moment. It made me realise how potentially devastating a small error can be in our job. This scared the hell out of me. Making doctors and nurses work twenty-four hours on the trot as we were doing at the time was crazy and dangerous. Especially for the poor patients coming in for an operation/emergency during the final, and most exhausting hours of our shift.

The doctor, in this case, was very understanding, if a little miffed, and the patient was fine. But from then on, I always asked everyone to repeat stuff at least twice over the phone for *la rosbif*. I'm naturally pessimistic, so for me anticipation has become my number one priority at work. Being an anaesthetist is like flying a plane: double-check *everything* before taking off, and you're less likely to crash.

I eventually earned myself a new nickname with the arrival of a fresh intake of students who replaced our *promo* (set). It came from Emanuel, an adorable doctor who loved to tease me. We called him Manu for short. *Supermanu* when it came to handling emergencies.

"Ha!" he said, cackling to himself. "Now the fresh fish has arrived, nobody will be interested in our little, blonde Breetish nurse… you've passed your sell-by date, old girl! You are finished."

"Well," I huffed back. "What's the famous saying in

France? You make the tastiest soup in *la plus vieille* (the oldest) *marmotte!*"

I'd meant to say *marmite,* which is a big cooking pot. Of course, like the picture on a pot of marmite! I should have known that. A *marmotte*, however, is a small, stupid-looking creature with buck teeth that lives in the mountains and spends its time either sleeping or screeching its head off. I was now officially our department of anaesthesia's "old *marmotte*".

And the name stuck.

One of the best things about qualifying and working in the *déchocage* is that they give you a beep. A beep means that you are uber-important because you must be reachable at *all* times. Only the chosen few get to wear these little devices, transforming them into hospital VIPs. Mobile phones were still a relatively new gimmick, so hardly any of us had one. Even when on the toilet, in the shower or asleep in bed, maintaining contact with us was vital for the continued wellbeing of our patients, the community… in fact, humanity as a whole. At least we beep holders saw it as such.

On the rare occurrence that your beep actually beeps, you pray that it's in front of non-beep holders, showing off just how paramount you are. More often than not, we got beeped to replace a bored colleague who needed a pee. Or to fetch him/her a coffee.

I did, though, get beeped one morning for a real reason. Dragon was coming in with a twenty-year-old victim of a gunshot wound to the heart (very rare in this neck of the woods, unlike my old days in Manhatten). The patient was very unstable, Glasgow 3, blood pressure 70/30, heart rate high at 160/minute.

Not looking good.

We got him on the stretcher in the *déchocage* unit; X-rays immediately showed a bullet lodged in the left ventricle (the largest of the heart chambers). The most important thing at this stage was to open his thorax, try and get the bullet out and stop the bleeding.

His heart stopped beating at this point, and my colleague started cardiac massage. He had already been intubated at the scene. My job was to help put an arterial line into his radial artery, which gives a more accurate and continuous blood pressure reading. The reading was nearing zero; his chances of survival were not outstanding. We tried shocking him twice without success. We hooked up a super-fast blood transfusion and adrenaline pump.

The cardiac team were waiting in theatre, and we ran there with the stretcher as fast as we could. The surgeon was scrubbed and ready. Rather than waste time disinfecting and drying the thoracic skin with swabs as usual, seeing that the situation was so urgent, he instructed the theatre scrub nurse to just chuck the bottle of alcohol and iodine mixture over the patient's chest before taking his electric saw to cut through the sternum.

Suddenly, it was bonfire night. The patient exploded into flames. The mixture of alcohol, oxygen and electricity had made a scout's marshmallow of our patient's operating table.

Luckily, the damage was more burnt foam than flesh, and the young man actually survived the ordeal. It's incredible how often this happens. Not even counting Gitane-puffing surgeons and alcohol-based disinfectants, fires in the operating room can be caused by something as benign as patients not removing make-up or moisturising cream, which often contain paraffin.

I decided it was time for me to take some driving lessons. I hadn't driven more than a couple of times since I'd passed my test years ago in England, and having a baby in the car was making me increasingly safety conscious. Roundabouts in France were the real challenge; occasionally, in a moment of doubt, I just went *over* instead of around them. I'd also come face to face with a clanging, furious Grenoble tram just enough times to make me seriously question my ability to take the wheel. These were nothing, however, compared to the devastating results of patients involved in terrible road traffic accidents. I swore to myself that Alex would never own a motorbike; they always tended to come second place in a head-on collision with any other vehicle – notably lorries. Lorry driver patients who crossed my path in our *déchocage* tested positive for a multitude of illegal substances on a multitude of occasions.

The world championship medal for driving under the influence of alcohol has to go to a certain strawberry-nosed removal van employee at 400 milligrams per deciliter of blood. It's almost scientifically impossible to be alive in that state, never mind happily driving someone's furniture around the country. With all this churning around in my mind, I booked ten lessons with Madame Bottelli of the Bottelli driving school or *auto école*. Now, many, many ridiculous laws exist around the world, but the silliest law in the universe has to be *la priorité à droite*, priority to the right, in France. This allows a car that is chugging down a side road at the speed of Brian (the stoned snail from *The Magic Roundabout*) to come out and turn onto the main road (that you're hurtling along at 50mph) without having to stop! Thereby, in the best-case scenario, causing a screeching of brakes, a waving of arms and a long string of "*putains*!"

My new instructor showed me round the car, pointed out various pedals and buttons, then asked if I was familiar with the gears? Yes, actually. Quite intimately. The number of patients I'd seen admitted in A+E impaled onto gear sticks was astonishing. It was always the same story. "You'll never believe me nurse, but I was just moving over from the passenger side to the driver's seat, when I slipped."

The first lesson underway, Madame Bottelli actually seemed quite pleased with my driving which gave me a first fragment of confidence. I started to relax... and put my foot down a little harder on the accelerator. Having no knowledge at the time of the stupid *priorité à droite* rule, I then almost collided with a Renault Scenic, which had pulled out of a narrow road extremely slowly, to my right.

My instructor let out a strangled shriek as I skidded to a halt, and my natural, instinctive reaction was to do what any English person would have done in that situation: I scowled at the other driver and stuck two fingers up at him. Surprisingly, he just smiled, waved and drove off. Hmm… in my experience, the French weren't the forgiving type. Something was amiss.

Madame Bottelli looked at me out of the corner of her eye. "Vat vas *zat?*" she asked, motioning to my hand.

"*Pardonnez-moi,*" I explained. "It's a silly thing from back home. This is how we tell someone that we're, well, not very *happy* with them."

"In zis country, we only use *one* finger. Ze middle one." She showed me. "Zat stupide driver sinks you gave him ze piss sign." She turned in her seat to look at me. "In ze car, we are not at piss, we are at war! You must beep your horn *much* more often. You're in France now, *bon Dieu*! For God's sake!"

There is a questionable myth that during the Hundred Years' War, English archers' right fore and middle fingers were chopped off by the French (yes, them again) when captured, thus preventing the now three-fingered English archer from holding a bow and arrow. Therefore, whenever a Brit wanted to tease the French enemy, they held up these two fingers in the air as a gesture of mocking defiance. The same legendary insult has continued up to the present day.

Where the single-finger variety comes from, I have no idea.

I personally found fifty euros an hour quite a hefty fee for teaching insults, although they did come in handy. I henceforth bombed around like Starsky in my Fiat Uno, honking furiously and showing my middle finger to anyone who waited for a nanosecond too long for the lights to change to green. I was really starting to blend in.

During the time that I was working in Grenoble, a new *ministre de l'intérieur* (home secretary) was appointed: a short, agitated man named Nicholas Sarkozy. He was making a rather unfortunate name for himself, both by wearing ridiculous shoe insteps but also by imposing speed cameras around the country's highways and byways. This was an extremely unpopular decision. The French hate being told what to do – especially in a car.

But, as someone working in *déchocage*, dealing with the effects of road traffic accidents on an almost daily basis, the result was remarkable. My colleagues and I had less stressful days, more time to deal with other patients, and there were fewer bed shortages in intensive care. Not to mention the economic and ecological advantages of sending the Dragon and SAMU teams out less often.

We witnessed first-hand the real consequences that a political decision can have at ground level.

One of the bonuses of working at the big city hospital was that it could get you out of a scrape with *les flics* (the local police). With my newfound confidence in a car and Madame Bottelli's words of wisdom, despite Mr Sarkozy's efforts, I was now driving like one of the natives.

One sunny afternoon, I was heading over to Christine's house in Eybens. The traffic lights were just turning orange, but I raced through them, which was, all things considered, a particularly stupid thing to have done. Blue lights started flashing behind me almost immediately, and a man's voice told me to pull over through an embarrassingly loud loudspeaker. *Shit, shit and merde.*

"*Bonjour, officer!*" I said with a wide-eyed innocent smile, winding down the window. "*Il y a un problème?*"

He asked for my papers. My nurse's badge was sticking out

next to the driving licence in my purse.

"*Vous travaillez au CHU! Vous êtes infirmière?*" (You're a nurse at the CHU?)

I nodded in the affirmative.

"*Vous allez où?*" (Where are you going?)

Since I couldn't beat them, I decided to simply lie through my teeth.

"There's an emergency liver transplant. They're waiting for me in theatre."

He looked impressed. What a mug. "*Suivez-nous.*" (Follow us.)

I had a full police escort to the hospital entrance! Lights, sirens and all. It was brilliant. I hid until they left, then drove off to tell Christine all about it.

Christine, in turn, told me about a run-in she'd had with the local *gendarmes*. Tom had been knocking back the beers one evening and insisted upon driving. They got into a fight about it, but he eventually persuaded her that he was sober enough. They started making their way slowly home from O'Callaghan's in their tattered old Peugeot, swerving all over the road.

A *gendarmerie* van stopped the car halfway along the quay, instructing them to turn off the engine and wind down the driver's side window for an alcohol breathalyser test. Amazingly, it was negative. The surprised *flics* ushered them on their way.

How was that possible? The car was British: a left-hand drive. They'd breathalysed Christine, the sober *passenger,* by mistake.

As I emerged from the fog of those early days of motherhood, after having enjoyed being pampered for six days in the hospital and being able to go back to work stress-free after finding a wonderful *nounou*, I reflected on the difference between French vs non-French offspring raising. For comparison, I had my

American, British and Belgian friends.

According to many people and much-published literature, French parents have better-behaved children, apparently for the simple reason that they put themselves first. They are not at the beck and call of their little loved ones and don't feel the slightest bit guilty about it. Some children even have to address mum and dad with *vous* instead of *tu*.

Their kids are, therefore, not necessarily at the epicentre of the universe, with all the other planets circling around them. They are not allowed in-between meal snacks, must sit straight at a desk even in the toddler class, and have to say "*Bonjour*" to every adult encountered on their path. Teachers don't sit reading stories on bean bags or give little Timmy a cuddle when he scrapes his knee. No, Timmy has to man up. There is a respectful distance and sharp telling off for any naughty behaviour. *Non* means non.

In the UK, I've noticed that "no" often means maybe… oh alright, go on then. Yes.

Chucking spaghetti and chicken nuggets around a restaurant and then hiding under the table to empty the saltshaker is a definite *non-non*. French children sit at the table mobile-phone-free, finish what's on their plate (even the strange organic green stuff, snails, frogs' legs etc.) and never interrupt adult conversations. And you can be reasonably sure that the spoiled brat screaming and running up and down the aisle of the train/plane/church because there's no Wi-Fi for its iPad is *not* a French one. Googoo gaagaa language certainly does not exist in France's baby world, either.

The differences in the way English and French children are raised extend to school too. French children are taught to read and write *comme il faut* with a proper fountain ink pen. At a young age, they invariably have joined-up writing, are able to tell the time and tie their own shoe laces. In fact, if they can't do any of these, they are seen to be somehow lacking. Schools appear to be generally so much more laid back in the UK, but conversely, there is much more helicopter-type obsessive parenting in Britain which I haven't yet encountered in France. In French schools, the names of each class are confusing enough – CM1, CP, CE2 – and then once they get to secondary school, everything goes backwards: *6ème, 5ème* all the way to *1ère*. Then it's something called *terminal*. Sounds depressing. At eighteen, they're supposed to get their BAC (baccalaureate) and, by this point, already know what they want to do for the rest of their lives. Music, art, theatre and sport are important in themselves but of little academic value in France. Maths and French are the most important subjects by far, but literature, history and general culture are paramount too, and the level is very high. Children study all subjects up to A-level, including philosophy.

There is a distinct lack of integration of children with disabilities into mainstream education in France. I have no idea how they are educated, but they seem to be hidden away, which, in my view, is much to the disadvantage of the rest of society. There seem to be many uncomfortable social issues and challenges in some of France's society – gay marriage, the LGBTQ movement, and racial issues are also still quite taboo.

Despite all of this, quality education is free and generally available to all from the age of three. Just about anyone who works hard can get their *baccalaureate;* GCSE and A-level equivalent. School days are long and serious. Classes start at 8.30 a.m. and go on until 4 p.m. or after, and there's always loads of homework. Private schools exist, but not at extortionate prices as in Britain or the United States. Schools were generally closed on Wednesdays and open on Saturdays instead when our children were small, the idea being they get a break mid-week. We poor parents who needed a lie-in on Saturday mornings got shafted on *that* particular decision.

In Britain and the US, the emphasis is on pulling the kids *up* (rather than pushing them *down,* as teachers in French schools can sometimes be seen to do.) Teamwork, art and sports are important. Children with physical or learning difficulties mingle with others. Music is essential too, which is maybe one of the reasons why the British are better at it! Perhaps a well-balanced mixture of *both* types of schooling would foster more open-minded, well-adjusted young adults to emerge from their years of childhood learning.

Grenoble, as I mentioned, was full of expats. I saw an English-speaking group for new mothers advertised in the local supermarket window, which I decided to pop along to one day. Perhaps I'd meet some fun people at Open House with whom I could compare birthing horror stories? Have a piss-take at France's expense? Laugh together about the dildo physiotherapy? Maybe organise exchange babysitting, or borrow some English DVDs?

I was greeted instead by a bunch of bored, rich, American green-tea-drinking housewives, who all had Brazilian live-in nannies. They had invented their own complicated, posh *franglais* cockney: "Oh God, Ana, do come and clear up the mess. The baby's thrown up on the Bernard!" (Bernard Tapis is a French millionaire and famous personality, someone who, co-incidentally, I was to meet later on in my nursing travels. *Tapis* is French for carpet.) These ladies organised trips to places like fine art galleries and a nearby glove factory. I preferred going for a walk or down the pub. We had absolutely nothing in common. So I left them to it.

Alex was growing and heading towards his first birthday. He was adorable, with his toothy grin, chubby tummy, blond hair and big blue eyes. He melted our hearts. But then everyone looks at their offspring through rose-coloured spectacles, don't they? Nobody sees a 'fugly' kid, as my paediatrician friend in the UK calls them, when they look at their own child. As someone once put it, children are like farts: the only ones you can put up with are your own.

You spend the first year of your children's lives willing them to walk and talk; these first word and first step moments are filmed, clapped and celebrated with champagne toasts. The next fifteen or so years are then spent telling them to sit the hell down and shut the hell up. In fact, looking after a small child is just like looking after a drunk friend at the end of a night out. You assist them into a sitting/standing position, gently coax them to drink some water, hold them as they stumble around and then take their clothes off before putting them into bed. They may pee and/or poop themselves. Helping to avoid them choking on their own vomit may be required. I'd had extensive training, both as a friend and a nurse. I was prepared. But still, it was exhausting.

We were, at last, getting to the stage where we could get a babysitter and start going back out to pubs, friends' houses and the cinema again. The cinema represented two hours of baby-free, popcorn-chomping escapism. Heaven! Plus, I had really begun to appreciate French movies.

In New York, Eddy and I had spent many a Monday night at the International Cinema on 21st Street. Monday was French night. I was pleasantly surprised by how much I loved these films, despite having to squint at the subtitles, and this soon became a weekly habit which we looked forward to with much glee and anticipation.

For people who haven't discovered this art form, because maybe like me, you equated French acting with their singing, prepare to stand corrected. As with all countries, they've made their share of rubbish. But, and indulge me here, I'd like to share a few of the best ones with you for any wannabe French film buffs out there. *Le Grand Bleu, Delicatessen, Ridicule, La Cage aux Folles, Les Visiteurs, Le Grand Vadrouille* and

Intouchables are really worth checking out. Watching these has filled my life with many happy hours.

Slowly then, nights out at the cinema became an option again. We threw in the odd trip to a restaurant, too. We were emerging from the sleepless nights with permanent suitcases under our eyes but nevertheless having regained some semblance of our previous adult life.

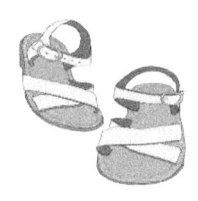

9. FROM THREE TO FOUR

Another baby, and a return home

So naturally, just as we were starting to get used to some long- awaited sleep and baby-free sanity, I got pregnant again.

A boy followed by a girl is known as *le choix du Roi* in France: the King's choice. Little Emilie came into the world two years after her brother. We had to choose names that were pronounceable and acceptable in both languages. Pippa was obviously out of the question. As were Fanny, Randy and Aurelie…

We thought she was totally amazing, the most beautiful baby girl ever born. Of course, looking back over the photos, we realise that she resembled a failed Russian experiment. A sort of beady-eyed potato. She's gorgeous now, which we're all mildly relieved about. I was just happy to have one of each; it meant I wasn't going to be asked to have any more.

Now that I had sweet little babies, my mother crawled out of the woodwork. She wasn't exactly Supernanny, but we were talking again, and she even came to visit. I'd hardly seen her since the wedding, which she'd done her best to sabotage. With her came news of my little brothers, now also uncles. I was over the moon to be in touch with them and hear that they were doing rather well after surviving all those years in Mum's "care". I decided to pay a visit to the UK in order to visit them.

Christophe willingly and selflessly took some time off

work, to give me a welcome break from the kids. I had been unbelievably homesick and found myself counting down the days (and sleepless nights) until I left.

It's funny the things you miss about Britain. You only realise these things even exist once you're gone. Number one is, of course, the food. I was gagging for an Indian takeaway, sticky toffee pudding and a proper Sunday roast. I'm not saying that French cuisine isn't wonderful; it is. But what you grow up surrounded by stays with you, infused into your brain and palate, influencing your judgement despite all things learned since. With a simple glance at a jar of Marmite or a sachet of butterscotch Angel Delight I salivate more than when presented with a more gastronomic *canard à l'orange, soufflé au chocolat* or *risotto aux truffes*. It's all very Pavlovian.

The weather in England *is* rather on the wet side. Our green and pleasant land is so green because it rains... and rains. And then rains some more. You only know it's summer because the rain is slightly warmer.

But then there are the people. The wonderful British public. What I love when I go home is the light, cheery street conversation, so lacking in Grenoble.

"Morning, love, alright?"

"You go ahead, sweetheart. I'm in no rush."

"See you again, babe, take care. Gawd bless!"

And this is all from complete strangers. I may be mistaking them for someone who actually gives a monkey's, but it's lovely to hear all the same.

Objectively, France is an astonishingly beautiful country. It has the stunning beaches of Corsica, the snow-capped Alpine peaks, the ancient Alsatian forests, the numerous mighty, stone-walled *châteaux* and the unique odour of pine trees, citrus fruits and Laurier bushes in the Provence region.

There are, for me, however, certain special places in the UK that are unbeatable when it comes to finding truly magical spots.

No image, dream or memory evokes feelings of peace in me quite like the forest at Sandringham. There's a reason why the Queen chose to live here for much of the time. Sandy paths run amongst the trees, daffodils and bluebells, spring sunlight rippling through them, casting tiny, moving shadows in front of each step you take, as butterflies dance and flicker.

The only sound is birdsong, buzzing and leaves fluttering in the gentle wind. The smell is pure Norfolk woodland: apple, lavender and wild grasses. Roses, brambles and blackberries add to the perfume as you pass by. If a fairy or unicorn were to cross my path, I wouldn't be at all surprised there! A simple stroll around Sandringham turns into an almost spiritual adventure. It's like walking through a Shakespearian sonnet.

The Mwnt beach at Ceredigion in Wales is so unspoilt and breathtaking that, for me, it beats anything that Corsica or even Crete can offer. Despite having a name impossible to pronounce, it is a gem of a place. A hidden cove of golden sand surrounded by dunes, upon which stands a whitewashed Celtic church, the only sign of human presence. Dolphins and porpoises frolic in the surrounding midnight-blue sea.

Obviously, you'll need to wear a wetsuit if you want to go swimming; temperatures on the Welsh coast are a long way from the Mediterranean. But watching the surfers and eating fresh fish 'n chips washed down with a local beer warms you up enough to forget that your fingers and toes have turned slightly numb.

Speaking of surfing, Cornwall, like Wales, has a unique cultural identity, so much so that it was granted status as having its very own ethnicity, recognised by the State in 2014. This particularity is felt in the landscapes, food and climate. Despite the busy seaside towns, there is a wildness about the place that I adore. Spectacular cliffs look down upon the rugged coastline and huge waves, where pirates once hid treasure in the coves along the sandy beaches.

A picnic of steaming Cornish pasties and local cider on

Porthcurno beach is unbeatable.

The Cotswolds are a long chain of hills starting from Bath in South West England and are described as a region of outstanding natural beauty. The rural way of life has been preserved in this unique, special place, where houses are built in golden, honey- coloured stone and surrounded by rolling green hills. Whenever I sing *Jerusalem* at a church wedding (William Blake's idea of heaven created in England, so legend has it), images of the Cotswolds come to mind.

There are many fine stately homes and magnificent old castles in Britain, but Chatsworth is my favourite. Set in expansive parkland, backed by the rocky hills of the glorious Peak District rising up to heather moorland, it is a truly original and awe-inspiring vision. The quality of the Baroque art and garden landscapes are unparalleled. The image of the great house mirrored onto the beautiful front lake is surely one of the world's most stunning and famous scenes. Lying on a blanket on the grounds reading *Pride and Prejudice* whilst munching on a slice of the famous regional Bakewell tart is the meaning of true happiness.

The Scottish Highlands are just as you've imagined in your dreams. The mist-covered lochs, ancient forests and abandoned ruins are simply mythical. Dark tales of clan battles, haunted castles and lake monsters are legendary. Perhaps it's because of my ancestors, but I have never encountered such a bewitching country. There is simply no comparison on earth to Scotland. One aches to behold such incredible and diverse beauty in the form of pure, raw, powerful nature. The 13th- century Eilean Donan Castle is the home of our Macrae clan. Situated on a tiny island at the meeting point of three great lochs, it is, to me, quite simply the most alluring place in the world.

All of these places I discovered with nursing friends. Either they had been born there, and we went to stay with their families, or we took vacations and long weekends together. If I hadn't chosen this career path, I doubt I would have dared venture very far from London.

I sorely missed our great British sense of humour, depicted on certain television programmes (thank goodness for satellites) such as *Fawlty Towers*, *Blackadder* and *Top Gear*. Or by comedians like Ricky Gervais, Michael Macintyre and my East End favourite, Mickey Flannagan.

Then there are the wonderful London museums that I visited so often as a child (because they were, and mostly still are, free). I especially loved the Natural History Museum; its enormous dinosaur, then blue whale reproduction in the great hall instigated my lifelong fascination with animals. Not forgetting the fabulous British, Victoria & Albert and Science Museums.

For lovers of art, you can amble around the Design Museum, The National Gallery and Tate Modern for hours of gaping wonder. And that's just in London. Although I have to admit that I don't always understand the extreme artistic value of some of the Tate's canvases; there's one that is just plain grey. It's called… *Grey*. Not very original. But worth millions! Maybe I could start painting *Yellow* and become stinking rich.

I missed it all, and I was very much looking forward to getting back home.

It was in this spirit of excited patriotism and general devoted Britishness that I arrived at Gatwick airport. I was even wearing a copy of my infamous magic Union Jack knickers. These were usually reserved for important international rugby games, as every time I remembered to wear them for a match, the England team would win. I eventually lost these original good luck charms when I catapulted them at Robbie Williams' surprised face from the front row during a concert in Lyon. Sorry about that, Robbie… they *were* clean. I promise.

Two identical handsome blond heads started shouting my

name as I wheeled my suitcase through Nothing to Declare. After much hugging and hair ruffling, we headed by taxi to a bar of their choosing. It was incredible how many years it had been since we'd seen each other, kept apart by our manipulative mother. We were so keen to catch up that everybody was shouting at once. The taxi driver looked terrified.

I learned that Tom, the eldest of the three, had gone on holiday to Thailand after graduating with a first-class honours degree in medieval history (his brilliant thesis described the grotesque medical consequences of prostitution in the 10th century) and had decided never to come back. Tom probably just wanted to get as far away from mum as possible. How he earned a living, they did not know.

We clambered out one by one onto the kerb at Wardour Street and entered the Village Soho bar. I was surprised to find myself the only female customer in there, but then I noticed that there were lots of male couples sitting around holding hands and snogging.

The penny dropped.

The boys then told me about their coming out experience with our mother. Apparently, she'd simply remarked, "You may as well go and hang yourselves now. Death from AIDS isn't pleasant." Good old Mum: you could always count on her for a bit of sensitivity, empathy and compassion when going through difficult times.

Although identical to look at, Roger and Chris couldn't have been more different in every other way. Roger was the academic boffin, specialising in all things Shakespearean. He'd gone as far as completing a PhD and had designed a 3D virtual reality tour of the famous Rose Theatre. He worked as a university theatre teacher.

"A real-life drama queen!" I sniggered, predictably.

Mild-mannered and quietly spoken, he was dressed in a casual jacket, corduroy trousers and trainers. Chris was more *street* smart. Having left school early, he'd worked his way up in the internet design world and was now an established leading player. All of Chris' clothes had Gucci or Adidas labels on them. His hair was tied back in a ponytail. He smoked, was loud, vivacious and liked to party.

We slowly filled in all the gaps: schooldays, work, relationships… so many missed shared experiences… but I got the feeling we were going to make up for lost time in the future. I told them about Christophe, Alex and Emilie, my anaesthesia job and the crazy French. They, in turn, recounted the difficult years with mum, dealing with all of her attempted suicides and embarrassing rages. They'd had a tough time.

We kept our meeting conspiratorially secret from her. Our childhoods had been hurtful and traumatic; we wanted a new beginning. A new togetherness.

As we later drove to Chris' home, I noticed the old 1970s ugly London tower blocks were being knocked down and replaced by flashy new high rises: triangular, box or cone-shaped in glistening silver and blue, powered by wind.

Chris had wisely invested in one of these new apartments. The price of his tiny one-bedroom flat would buy you a castle in *la Corrèze* region of France. We dropped my backpack off, our stomachs lurching in the speeding elevator. The view was spectacular – sparkly night-time London from twenty-five floors up with the Thames weaving its way towards the horizon, passing under all the landmark bridges.

After showering and changing, the three of us headed out again to the Fridge club, a converted cinema in Brixton.

It was Love Muscle Party night, one of the hottest gay spots in town. This was a slight change from Cinderella's, and it was fantastic. I had met lots of gay men both in Brighton and New York, always finding them to be full of life, fun and laughter. And usually *utter* bitches, too. We were still living in an era of renowned homophobia, but in this largely auto-segregated venue, they were really able to let loose.

I spotted Boy George, Marc Almond and George Micheal

all surrounded by starry-eyed shirtless hangers-on and Jamiroquai's Jay Kay dancing with an exquisite blonde. Soul 2 Soul often hosted, but tonight it was DJ Sophie (now Tallulah Goodtimes), a great friend of Chris', who was spinning the discs. The music was a fast-beat techno pop remixed with a little swing. I loved dancing amongst guys in wigs, heels and lipstick; people behaving just as they liked and not giving a hoot about what others may think. It was very different from France, where everyone always appeared to be extremely self- conscious and terrified of being judged.

Londoners, like New Yorkers, are free spirits. "We're not necessarily here for a *long* time… but we're gonna make sure it's a *good* time!" Chris shouted to me over the music and smoke.

I woke up on Chris's living room floor late on Saturday morning, more than a little hungover. I resembled a racoon with black make-up smudged all round my eyes. Luckily, I'd remembered to take two 500mg paracetamol tablets washed down with a litre of water before passing out. Nursing school teaches you a lot of important stuff.

For purely recuperative purposes, we ambled over to Elephant and Castle's Greasy Spoon Café for a proper English breakfast and a feast of weekend papers. By the time we left to catch the Brighton train, I was feeling right as rain. Chris had decided to accompany me to Brighton, having bought a property there, too. I had a rendezvous with Jo, Julia and Rob at a pizzeria near the Pavilion that evening. Chris and I said goodbye to Roger; he was heading back to Nottingham. He promised to come over and visit us soon. He wanted to introduce me to his partner: a brilliant engineer with whom he was planning to emigrate to Australia.

Itchy feet appeared to be a family trait.

Coming back to Brighton was such a thrill; my pulse quickened as we approached, just as it always had. There was still exactly the right balance of tacky seaside town, bourgeois elegance and mad, party ambience. After a quick stroll along the seafront, we trotted up North Street. I said goodbye to Chris, and I almost skipped up to India gate, where I had arranged to meet the others. I stopped dead in my tracks when I saw the whole nursing gang standing outside our old favourite Italian restaurant, glasses raised in hands!

Julia had decided to turn my visit into a reunion. Even our tutor, Julie, was there – and good old Dr Williams had turned up with his pregnant wife. It was he who offered to get the next round of drinks in. Being a doctor, he was probably the only one who could afford it; there were about twenty of us. In the old days, five quid used to suffice for an entire night out… now all it got you was a pint and a small packet of peanuts.

"I'll have a bottle of champagne, cheers, mate!" said Tiny Tim. "It's the least you owe me after all the drugs and prostitutes I supplied you with for the on-call room when you were a house officer." Mrs Williams stared at her husband open-mouthed in disgust. Huffily pulling her coat back on, she turned around and left, slamming the restaurant door… as raucous laughter exploded all around the table.

Julia had had two children by then and had married a hilarious copper: the laughing policeman, I call him. They were continuously taking the piss out of each other, the sign of a happy marriage. Julia was doing brilliantly as a head practice nurse, specialising in chronic pulmonary disorders.

Jo was pregnant with baby number three. She'd met her husband at the hospital when he'd come to visit his best mate, who had been admitted to her ward. They lived half of the time on the island of La Palma in the Canaries for his astronomy work. He's incredibly sweet, great for Jo, and, incidentally, one of the funniest people on earth. He always addresses me by my middle Scottish name for some strange reason.

"Rae, Rae, Rae… *what* have you been up to, *now*?" he'd ask, shaking his head in mortified disbelief.

They had beautiful children and complemented each other

perfectly. Jo worked at the local university in Sheffield when in the UK, looking after hundreds of students' various health matters.

Rob had, at last, settled down and was married to an adorable paediatrician, who, luckily, had forgiven me for the Calais escapade and shaved eyebrows on their wedding day. They were expecting their first baby, a little girl. He had undergone specialised training in intensive care and moved over to the John Radcliffe, Oxford's biggest teaching hospital. We laughed and reminisced about our nurse training, but I sensed he was calmer now and more peaceful. Some of us have to go through that crazy stage before we can just chill out with one special person.

Very few of the group were still in nursing, I was surprised to learn - disheartened by the poor pay and conditions, preferring to leave work to start a family or having found other professional paths to follow. These were the first accounts I heard of just how grim the NHS had become since I'd left England.

The next day, a few of us went for a walk across the downs to Devil's Dyke, finishing off a perfect weekend with a good old Sunday roast lunch in something called a *gastro* pub. I was a little worried. *Gastro* in French is short for gastroenteritis (gut rot), but luckily there were no dodgy tummy rumblings, despite an extra helping of sticky toffee pudding, and I was able to make the flight home on time, my suitcase stuffed to the brim with prawn cocktail crisps and marmite.

Now that I'd had my England fix, I was happy to be home, and the kids hadn't even starved to death. The house, however, *did* look like we'd been burgled at least twice.

Back at work, there was some good news. Christine had decided to change jobs and been hired as the new head nurse of our surgical unit. This meant that I was no longer the only *rosbif* in the place. Someone English to have lunch with at last! As we sometimes accompanied poorly patients after their surgery back to the wards, I'd often bump into her. It was nice to have someone to compare professional nursing life between France and the UK with. The differences are innumerable, and we spent hours mulling and giggling over them.

Pristine, modern French hospitals and throw-away paper trouser scrubs were a long way from old Victorian brick buildings and Nightingale wards with patients down each side. Not to mention capes, buckles and silly hats.

In the UK (and America), for example, leeches are often used in facial reconstruction surgery to absorb haematomas. We just couldn't imagine any prim French nurse putting her delicate little hand into a jar of *those* slimy creatures. I have to say that although I was taught how to apply them, I tend to agree with our continental colleagues in this instance. Every nurse has their limits.

We were surprised they'd never heard of the good old stool chart, either: Britain's nurses' famous legacy to poo! An interesting fact taught in nursing schools, for example, was that healthy poo sinks. If you have a floater, it may be a sign of nutrient malabsorption. If the stool does sink, but some of it sticks on the way down, well, that could be a diet too high in fat. Pale poo may indicate liver or gall bladder issues. Important stuff.

We chuckled at each other's vocabulary mishaps, too. Christine had been called to help with placing a nasogastric (NG) tube into a patient's nose. Her French was rather limited back then, even worse than mine. She just about knew the words for arms and legs, but a *nostril*? Not a clue.

"Bonjour, monsieur," she introduced herself, dangling the long, thin plastic tube at him. "*Je vais mettre ceci dans votre* I'm going to put this thing into your… um… *trou*?" Hole. As in *arse*-hole. The accompanying auxiliary had to immediately vacate the room and could be heard howling with laughter in the corridor.

Christine and I found ourselves in most need at the hospital during the winter months. Brits descend on the Alps in great numbers during the ski season, the only problem being that very few of them actually know how to ski. The main medical presenting problems are not always trauma-based but regularly alcohol-related. That and hypothermia brought about from skiing naked.

One guy from Birmingham was extremely happy to see us; people who could actually understand him at last! This one had been hospitalised with two badly fractured legs, the result of "sledging" down a mountainside on a plastic bin bag. He had obviously been immobilised, meaning that any urinating would now need to be done in a special hand-held receptacle.

"I keep asking them for a *bottle*... but they just keep bringing me bloody *wine*!" He moaned in a Brummie accent, clutching his lower abdomen. "I'm *bursting*!" As I said before, booze can be had on prescription.

"I'll go and find what you need," said Christine, running off to fetch the long, white object of desire. She was back within no time.

"Here's a *pistolet*," she said to the patient, handing it to him. *Pistolet* is indeed the French word for urinal... but it is also the translation for a gun. He seemed to be familiar with only the latter. "And what the hell am I supposed to do with *that*?" He shouted after her, wiggling the plastic contraption in the air.

"*Shoot* me bloody self?"

O'Callaghan's was still our place of choice to unwind in the evening. The girls' new game was explaining to someone French that the diminutive of the British name Richard was Dick. And then the conversation progressed to: "So, any Dicks in your family? Oh, there is one! Is he nice? Oh, so you like Dick, do you…?" Etc. Etc.

There was a new barman. The old one was in the hospital. (I'd seen his name on the liver transplant waiting list.) The four of us walked up to order drinks.

"Is your name Richard, by any chance?" We asked sniggering childishly.

"*Bah, non,*" he said. "Eet's Mustafa."

"Oooh." Temporary disappointment.

"Then I Must… afa beer, please!"

"Mustafa rum and coke, me!"

"Mustafa box of matches."

"Mustafa packet of crisps, too…"

The long winter evenings flew by. We thought we were so funny. I don't think Mustafa agreed.

Our other favourite game was pretending to ask an unsuspecting French person the time. We'd go up to random men, frowning quizzically whilst pointing at our watches and say, "Excuse me, please. Do you have a big pair of hairy bollocks?"

"Yes, yes I do… *bien sûr.* Of course!" They'd charmingly inform us. "Alf past eight."

Stupid? Absolutely. Made us cackle like a coven of witches, though.

Christophe's announcement when I got home later that particular evening wiped the silly smile off my face. His company had bought a subsidiary based in the Yvelines (a region to the west of Paris). They wanted him to head the finance team from there. The old *marmotte* was on the move again.

I cried on my last day at work. I'd grown to love the

extraordinary anaesthesia and surgical teams at Grenoble. We were like one massive family. We often spent more time with each other than with our own kin.

Here's just one story that will give you an idea of how special and amazing those people are and the incredible work that is done at the CHU. Many of our *déchocage* patients were admitted somewhere between life and death… some spoke of seeing a light and being enveloped in a feeling of warmth and peace before we brought them back from the brink. We were all interested in the subject of near-death experiences. Everyone is spiritually curious to some degree, after all.

One of the anaesthesia house officers had the idea of writing a word on top of the round operating lights. This involved climbing up high on a ladder, making the word impossible to see by anyone on the ground. You'd literally have to levitate to the ceiling to be able to read it, and what had been written was kept top secret.

This house officer asked us to listen for any abstract words which patients might mention, having experienced and survived cardiac arrest. One man, victim of a huge gastrointestinal bleed, regained consciousness when his heart began beating again following a life-saving blood transfusion, cardiac massage and defibrillation.

"*H… hippopotame.* Hippopotamus," he whispered as soon as the breathing tube was removed.

Weird, I thought.

"Hey, Martin!" I said to the house officer the next time I saw him. "What was the word up on the light? You can tell me; I'm leaving. We'll probably never see each other again."

You guessed it.

Hippopotame.

The team laid on a special goodbye breakfast a n d then gave me my choice of operating room as a treat for my final shift. I chose my favourite: cardiothoracic. I knew everyone in the room except the *perfusionist*, who was new. I got chatting with him, and he told me a story about his last workplace at a CHU in the north of France.

When a patient has cardiac surgery, they're generally put on a pump which bypasses their own circulation. The blood is shunted outside the body and oxygenated through a machine so that the surgeon can get the painstaking work done on a non-beating heart. The person in charge of the pump is called a *perfusionist*.

One of the most important things that he or she needs to do is make sure all the various tubes are clamped and unclamped at the right moments. The one in the story hadn't yet mastered the whole *un*clamping part, unfortunately. There was a sudden buzzing and ringing of alarms as the pressure in the system hit overdrive. He felt the warm, sticky explosion before hearing it. The patient, mercifully, came away unharmed thanks to a massive, slightly panicked blood transfusion. According to this *perfusionist*, you saw the operating room windows turn red for miles around.

Already feeling nostalgic, we stuffed first our belongings, then our children, into the Fiat. Christophe took the wheel and headed north. I sat brooding, stroking our overweight guinea pig, Obelix, on my lap, watching as the now familiar mountains grew smaller and smaller in the wing mirror… until eventually flattening out under a dusky sky.

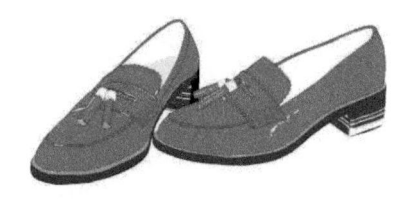

10. BACK TO PAREE

Mismanaging the stars

We decided to stop renting and buy our first house. The price per square metre in Paris *intra muros* (within the city walls) meant we had to look a bit further away. Parisian, like London, house prices are exorbitant.

The *Yvelines* is a particularly pretty, leafy *département* of France, being largely covered by forests. It's only half an hour's drive into the city and, when we were looking, prices were affordable for young couples such as us. After many visits, we settled on a small, semi-detached house in Orgeval, a pretty village not far from St Germain-en-Laye. It had a lovely garden and was a two-minute walk from the local school.

Once that was settled, I had to decide where to apply for my next job. The possibilities in Paris were endless – an exciting prospect. I was spoiled for choice in the country's capital, which was humming with hospitals. I worked a few CDDs, whilst updating and sending out my CV with something more permanent in mind.

A renowned international establishment caught my eye – a blissful nirvana (I imagined) where I would be surrounded by lovely Englishness. I applied, was called for an interview and was told that the doctors liked doing all the anaesthetic work themselves. No way were they going to share their extortionate salaries with a nurse. They just used a passing porter to hold the oxygen mask on the patient's face while putting in the IV – a much simpler, cheaper solution.

However, would I be interested in a *management* post?

I'd never thought about it. But why not? To me, management meant being in a position to help change things for the better. I had been impressed with their hiring procedure: each candidate had to pass a test on drug and calculation knowledge. The questions were well thought out and intended to weed out any potentially dangerous nurses. I have to say this was ingenious and a really good quality control initiative, even though, ideally, it shouldn't be necessary.

The salary they offered was surprisingly low for such a luxurious private hospital. Maybe that's normal, I told myself. Perhaps you get a bonus depending on your performance.

I had a niggling bad feeling about the place in the pit of my stomach but stupidly decided to ignore my instinct and accepted the offer to take charge of two, large post- operative recovery rooms. I was initially seduced by the international patients and personnel, as well as the fancy carpeted staff restaurant serving smoked salmon with foie gras and fig jam. Plus, of course, there was the constant possibility of bumping into Brad Pitt in the corridor. Any nurse would find *that* tempting, even the male ones.

From my new office window, I had a fortunate view of the car park. On my first morning at work, I spotted a dog suffocating inside a dark Audi sedan. The car windows were firmly closed on an extremely hot day, and it was stuck inside, trying to yelp for help through the misted-up glass. I love dogs, so I grabbed the nearest nurse, and we ran down the fire escape to the rescue. We managed to smash the back window open, get the poor thing out and resuscitate it. It must have been 50° inside the vehicle. Dogs are surprisingly easy to intubate, and as soon it got some oxygen and cool IV fluids on board, the animal was right as rain.

The dog's owner was extremely embarrassed and even offered an extensive thank-you contribution to the hospital's charity fund. (Although this *can* be tax deductible before you clap too soon.) He didn't even complain about his broken window to the director, luckily. That would *not* have gone down well on my first day. But I should have seen it as a sign.

From my privileged car-park view position, I got to see the glitterati arriving first-hand. Staff were forever barging into my room to take a peek at whichever star was climbing out of whatever Maserati, Porsche or black-tinted Mercedes that had just pulled up.

One day, my office was so heaving with people that I was pushed away from my desk by the mob and ended up falling off my chair. They were all screaming, "*Johnny! Johnny!*" like a bunch of lunatics.

"Who the hell's Johnny?" I asked, picking myself up off the floor.

Johnny Hallyday, I later learned, was France's biggest rockstar, worshipped and adored by millions. Girls were fainting over my desk… I had absolutely *no* idea what he even looked like.

This lack of popular cultural knowledge got me into trouble more than once. I was called to deal with a kerfuffle one day outside the larger recovery room doors, which can only be opened with a special badge. There was a gentleman making a hell of a fuss because he couldn't get in. He was insisting very loudly on being able to visit a family member inside.

I calmly explained to him that the person concerned was fine, but the anaesthetic team were in the middle of dealing with a complicated paediatric post-surgical incident, and it would be best not to disturb them. I told him that I could take a message to his kin, and he would be allowed in as soon as they were done. It didn't work; he just got louder, ruder and redder. My French wasn't up to that level of arguing, and this guy, as I found out later, was used to yelling orders at one of France's top football clubs all day.

Undeterred, he became more and more hostile, obviously used to getting his own way. He was really starting to piss me off. We were almost nose to nose, eyes unblinking, arms folded and hissing at each other like a couple of angry cats.

"*Laissez-moi entrer*!" Let me in!

"N.O.N."

"*Vous savez qui je suis?*" Do you know who I am?

"You must be mistaking me for someone who gives a *merde*."

This could have gone on forever, but there was no *way* he could win; I held the magic badge. Ha! Eventually, he gave in and wandered off, occasionally looking back at me with furrowed eyebrows, cursing and muttering under his breath.

There was hell to pay from my boss. He'd made an official complaint. Did I realise who I'd just offended so tactlessly? Well, in fact… *non*.

Just monsieur Tapis, an extremely famous French businessman, politician, millionaire football club owner, actor, singer and TV host who made regular charitable donations to the hospital.

Oops. Double *merde*.

Sometimes, even recognisable famous stars don't look at all like you imagine.

I entered the hospital lift one morning and came face to face with a long-haired man in slightly bedraggled clothes wearing round, blue sunglasses and smelling strongly of roll-ups. The head of security, who was next to me, reached for his phone. I imagined it was to call for backup in order to vacate this vagabond from the premises. He was quite a tough-looking fellow and didn't seem like he'd be easy to chuck out. I moved into the far corner, pretending to examine the buttons.

It was only when the lift opened at the maternity wing that it dawned on me.

"Security calling. Mr Depp is at level three, clear the way. Over."

"This way, please, sir," someone said, holding the lift doors open as I stepped out of the way sheepishly.

Mr Depp certainly left his mark on the hospital in his unique, original way. Hanging out of the window by his feet with a knife between his teeth, pirate style, he carved the name of his newborn daughter into the orange brick wall. Whenever friends came to visit me at work, I'd sneak them up and smugly show them the famous etchings. They were *well* impressed, I can tell you.

To be honest, I found managing people difficult. Especially French twenty-something-year-olds who were interested in anything *but* work. The number of *arrêt maladies* (sick days) was incredible – by British stiff-upper-lip-keep-on-going-whatever-happens standards, anyway. Not having been born yesterday, I could see very well that they were far from sick. Unless, that was, you counted hangovers.

"I need Tuesday afternoon off. It's for my yoga class, madame."

"Sorry, Adeline. I need you on Tuesday. I can't find a replacement so soon."

Tuesday comes, and guess what? Surprise, surprise… Adeline's got food poisoning and can't come in. We all ate the same thing at the cafeteria the day before, and no one else was unwell. Funny that.

Most of my day was subsequently taken up with the intense monotony of desperately trying to replace people at the last minute. Sometimes that person simply had to be me, in a desert of temporary nursing staff. It was all rather boring and frustrating. I wasn't happy and began to question if I was right for the job. My boss was a control freak and didn't allow me the slightest autonomy or to get involved in any of the more interesting projects. Bosses sometimes don't want to share their power for fear of being overturned. But she had nothing to fear from me.

"…I am incapable of channelling all your energee. You 'ave too much!" she told me, throwing her hands up in the air, exasperated. Only in France could having *too* much energy at work be considered a problem.

Uber-rich Emirates, Israelis, royalty, politicians and film stars came from all over the world in their private jets to be looked after by our famous doctors. They were capable of calling for a nurse to raise or lower the window blind by one centimetre. Or order caviar and a bowl of truffle soup at *exactly* 37°C. Or to insist on speaking to their unfortunate surgeon at 5 a.m. For the fifteenth time. On a Sunday.

There were several VIP suites where extra-wealthy customers could house family, friends, mistresses and private chefs. If one of these patients buzzed for a 1972 chilled Dom Perignon and a high-class call girl at midnight, well, someone made damn sure they got it.

These people were used to displaying this kind of behaviour, I suppose… but refusing to be looked after by someone of a certain race, insisting on being surrounded by hundreds of hazardous candles because they're a princess… or wanting to be anesthetised in their bedroom because they're scared of operating theatres overstepped ethical boundaries, as far as I was concerned. Perhaps it was my imagination, but it would seem that money *can* buy anything, and dubious practice hung like a dark cloud over the place.

I encountered some wonderful staff, but I never integrated well. I simply didn't fit in. It's a shame, really. The hospital collects huge donations from the rich, which enables it to be on the cutting edge of technology, research and medical equipment, making it a potentially highly exciting place to work.

There were regular rumours of political shenanigans. One day I remember getting to work only to look up and see a bunch of snipers crouching on the roof. When I asked what they were doing there, someone informed me that Fidel Castro had been admitted as a patient.

Now, hang on a minute. This hospital is full of foreigners, notably Americans. As in the people who tried to have the Cuban communist pro-Russian revolutionary leader assassinated in the 1960s. And now they're looking after the guy? Maybe the idea was to *take care* of him whilst taking care of him?

But then, just as unlikely was Osama Bin Laden's mother having a medical check-up there just hours before 9/11. And *that*, I found out, was confirmed by the world's media.

By pure luck, a headhunter contacted me around this time with a job. It was quite far away, on the southern outskirts of Paris, but I decided to go for the interview anyway. They were looking for someone to head recovery and help out in the anaesthetics department. The successful candidate would be expected to follow a managerial part-time master's degree.

It was thus in this underprivileged, colourful, multicultural Parisian suburb that I found professional utopia. The human resources director met me in the car park. Amel put the *human* back into resources. We walked down the road to the hospital. What a difference from the perfect, sterile 16th *arrondissement*. We passed homeless people sitting on their handmade cardboard beds. Amel knew all their names and stopped to chat. Yes, she would ask about a job in the kitchen, of course. As soon as a porter's position became available, she'd let the person know. If they needed any health advice or free vaccinations, she told them to go to the emergency room and give them her name. Did anyone require food or a safe place to sleep?

I was in the presence of greatness. A true saint. Few people have ever made such an immediate impression on me.

Kindness attracts kindness, as I was about to find out; the onsite team were amazing. Many of the doctors had names I had already heard of, being closely affiliated with the SFAR (Société Française d'Anesthésie et Réanimation).

The SFAR aims to improve anaesthetic practice by implementing and evaluating extensive national and international research. It is the stone onto which French anaesthesia is carved. Thousands of doctors and nurses hoard into Paris like sheep once a year for the famous four-day-long congress in September at Porte Maillot near La Place de L'Étoile.

There's even a medical congress joke:

Two doctors meet in the amphitheatre: a man and a woman. They get on really well, have dinner and drinks after the presentations, and then decide to spend the night together in a hotel.

The next morning, the man asks her, "Are you a surgeon by any chance? I'm only saying because you've scrubbed your hands clean at least twenty times since we met."

"Yes," she replies. "Orthopaedics, actually. And you? Are you an anaesthetist perhaps?"

"I am. How did you guess?"

"Easy… I didn't feel a thing!"

There were also several people very much involved in humanitarian charities. This hospital was regularly classed amongst the best French private healthcare institutions by the prestigious magazine *Le Point*.

When I met the large recovery team, they seemed more than competent but somewhat low on morale. Motivation needed a little stimulating, Amel told me. If I accepted the post, it was *carte blanche,* a blank cheque, to rally the troops.

I looked around me. The recovery room was huge enough to hold forty beds, with numerous floor-to-ceiling windows which were all shut and blocked. So, the gang worked permanently under artificial neon tubes. I knew that being exposed to daylight correlated to having more energy and, essentially, being in a better mood.

They're blocked from the outside, I was informed. We were five floors up, so there was no easy way of getting the mechanical shutters open. The window technician had apparently "forgotten" when they'd opened the hospital several years before. I pictured Manuel from Fawlty Towers with a screwdriver in his hand, scratching his head.

This was a Wednesday, which was paediatric surgery time on the school-free day of the week. The place was full of screaming kids. The noise was deafening. They were placed randomly in between adult patients in cots with high metal bars. Many had blood-splattered chins and gowns, the result of numerous tonsillectomies and adenoidectomies. They looked like wild caged animals.

A plan was sewing its seeds in my brain. "Ok," I said to Amel, "I'm in. But on two conditions…"

A few weeks later, I was packing up my old office to leave when, looking out of the window, I noticed two men with balaclavas over their heads running from the car park out into the main road towards a waiting car. They bundled in and screeched off. I immediately called security, but it was too late. They had made off with the hospital safe and tied up the security guard, who was found shocked but unharmed. I heard faint sirens, but I don't believe they were ever caught. With all the payments that were made in cash, I can only imagine how much money was stashed away in that big metal box. Perhaps enough for the villains to come back and get penis enlargements in here one day, I reflected.

I'd seen more male porn stars limping around with huge bandages swinging between their legs in those few months than I'd had *foie gras* sandwiches. This expensive and painful procedure involved injecting fat, taken from plumper parts elsewhere on the body, into the family jewels. Apparently, this makes the object of the camera more appealing for films and photo shoots.

Perhaps my idea of what makes an aesthetically pleasing picture differs from most.

In the city of Paris and its immediate surrounding area - *la région parisienne* - any non-Parisians are looked down upon as *ploucs*, which basically translates as peasants. We had accordingly changed out of our Grenoble country-bumpkin ways and muddy wellies back into smart suits, cocktail dresses and suede pumps.

They even speak differently in Paris. *Oui* is pronounced w*aaaay*, a longer, more condescending version of the original. But their haughty superiority did not stop the *la bourgeoisie* from shoving unlikely objects up their back passages, like everyone else.

I had only been in the new job a few days before a patient presented for theatre with a shower head lodged inside him. The *entire* thing. You must admire his determination, I suppose; it defied probability. Not to mention gravity.

We asked the usual questions of what, where, when, how and above all, why? But there, he cowered. Not another word passed his lips. Aha! The old Fifth Amendment approach.

"Oh, come on," I said. "I've seen it all before. You can trust me, I'm a *nurse*!"

After much gentle persuasion, it turns out he was "curious". And that's all he would say. Now don't get me wrong, curious is good. I wonder about a lot of things myself: Where do we come from? Why are we here? Is there life after death? Etc. But… what does a shower head feel like up my bum? Nope, that's not a question I've ever been particularly inquisitive about finding the answer to. Maybe I'm missing out on something amazing. We're not here to judge.

Something I did wonder about, however, is how I'd react if I came face to face with one of these patients at a dinner party one evening. *What* on earth would I say?

"Bonjour, madame! I look familiar? Yes… I sedated you whilst we pulled three golf balls out of your vagina. Or was it four, I'm not sure?"

"Enchanté monsieur, yes we have met before, actually. So, did that Eiffel tower come out of your anus in one piece?"

I'd make damn sure any pets were safely hidden away.

Dinner parties where the majority of the guests hail from a medical background should be avoided by the squeamish non-medical community. A tough demeanour (not to mention stomach) is required in order to make it through to cheese and dessert. The conversation ultimately turns into a contest of who's extracted the most memorable or exotic thing out of someone.

I think the prize must go to a young A & E doctor I met from Caen. He told me about a man who had found a WW2 bombshell whilst walking along the landing beaches of Normandy and decided to take his new toy home to play with. Later, when he inevitably arrived at the hospital emergency room, it was discovered that there was a risk the bomb may still be live. The military was called, and the patient was suddenly surrounded by a special squad unit in full armour, accompanied by dogs and robots. Not to mention cameras. Any hopes of passing incognito were dashed.

I made several simple changes to the recovery room, which revolutionised the workplace, and all at very little cost. The window blinds were lifted away using cranes. For the first time in years, there was daylight and sunshine in the air. We cracked open a couple of bottles of champagne to celebrate. At the end of the shift, of course!

Secondly, I created a paediatric space away from the adult patients. This area had toys (disinfected regularly) and comfy chairs so that the parents could be present for cuddles, along with television screens showing old black and white cartoons. The result was a decrease in post-operative pain medication consumption and, more importantly, screaming levels. The team were thus more relaxed, along with our adult patients, and those who preferred to look solely after children were assigned to this wing after receiving special training. All was quiet on the front again. The little monsters just needed a bit of segregation, attention and distraction.

Lastly, I gave up my lunch hour to do regular teaching sessions. For anyone interested in learning how a ventilator worked, anaesthesia pharmacology or reading ECGs, I made myself available at midday. The only thing that nurses appreciate more than free opportunities to extend their knowledge is a simple "thank you" at the end of their shift. A couple of cheap, uncomplicated, effective moves and I was rewarded by a significant drop in sick leave and a better overall ambience.

I remember one midday teaching the lunch-bunch about certain medications that can be passed directly down the intubation tube into the lungs – adrenaline, for example.

"Let's try it on, Annie, shall we? Give her a milligram."

One particularly enthusiastic young nurse immediately chucked a phial of adrenaline straight down Annie's throat.

(You are supposed to draw it up in a syringe first, then squirt it down the tube.) Not only was poor Annie having an acute myocardial infarction, but now her trachea was obstructed with broken glass.

Luckily Annie was just a dummy. We fished it out.

The team were happy, the patients were happy (apart from Annie, perhaps), the director was happy, and I was in hospital heaven.

At the same time, I had to embark on my own new educational adventure: a master's degree in health management, far over on the other side of Paris. Twice a week, I needed to be up at 4.30 in the morning in order to make the trip. I wasn't enthralled by the subject matter. Political science and accounting are not my things. It didn't help that many of the teaching staff were potty, radicalized Marxists.

What I *did* enjoy was the legal part. We studied numerous laws and cases. Nurses and doctors must have a minimum number of hours between shifts; this was an enlightening one. I realised that making someone work till 10 p.m. and then at 6 a.m. again the next day was illegal. So I changed the off-duty rota accordingly. Many managers do not, being understaffed and unable to find solutions. And, well, nobody ever gets caught, do they?

Healthcare establishment law is complex but logical. I like logic. In France, civil law is guided, page after page, by a book called *le Code Civil*, which was originally signed by Napoleon Bonaparte in 1804. They still use it to this day.

Public and private hospitals each have their own rules. A new law that intended to revamp the health system was about to be announced by Nicholas Sarkozy's government called HPST (Hôpital, Patient, Santé et Territoire). They were to introduce new regional governing bodies called the *Agences Régionales de Santé*, or ARS (that made me laugh out loud). Some of the ideas were positive, with an emphasis on disease prevention amongst minors, paying doctors a higher wage to set up in rural areas, more funding for cancer and co-operation between the private and public sectors.

But the essential problems of the *numerus clausus*[3] and nurses' pay/conditions were not addressed, as per usual. Giving total power to each hospital director was one of the more dreadful measures, in my opinion. There are good directors and not-so-good directors, after all. I worked with one who used to manage prisons. The problem was he still thought he was running a prison full of prisoners, not a hospital full of patients.

In any case, it was fascinating to study. I reasoned that the only way to make a real difference was through fighting for better rights via the unions and courts and studying hard in order to reach a position where you can make changes come about. Oh, and using one's vote. Wisely.

Speaking of voting, politics were a big part of our daily lives; French people talk about it *all* the time. Political debates were far more popular on evening TV than films and soap operas. There seemed to be a worrying uprising of extremist parties all over Europe. There were unsettling mumblings in the British parliament about wanting to leave Europe, too. I decided that I wanted to have my say in the next local and general elections. And stay European.

"Well then," Christophe said, looking up from *Le Figaro* with a smirk. "You'll have to get French nationality, won't you? Ha! My *rosbif* will become a Froggie!"

Putain. He was right.

---

[3] The *numerus clausus* (Latin for "limited number") was implemented to restrict admission of medical students into their second year because there were more applicants than available places.

I'd avoided the subject up till now for the simple reason that I just couldn't be bothered. It was like getting married all over again. The official government website, designed to help, simply tricked you into believing that it was a quick and easy procedure. Of course, once you'd paid the initial fee and reality was unveiled, the interminable tasks ahead started looming up like Mount Everest. As with all French bureaucracy, nothing is as it seems.

Firstly, you had to fill a load of stuff out online, including paying a tax duty. They then gave you an address to contact. There was no phone number. I checked over and over again and even physically drove around trying to locate it, but the address was non-existent.

Hitting a brick wall so soon into the procedure was demoralising, but thank heaven, there were blogs to help, written by innumerable souls who had been in the same sticky situation. Go to the *Mairie*, I was told; they are obliged to provide you with the magic phone number. It turned out, apparently, that they organised this little run-around on purpose to deter the less motivated due to a high demand for French identity and "a lack of town hall staff."

Having, at last, contacted the immigration team, I was given a long list of documents to send in, translated into French, of course, at a ridiculous cost by someone totally overbooked, named by them. It was a nightmare; I had to go back three times because of a missing page, misunderstanding, typo or new policy. "Oh, that's been changed since last month, didn't anyone tell you? I know it's written mother's birth certificate, but it's actually your father's that we need…"

And two months later, "Here's my father's original birth certificate. Is the dossier complete now?"

"Computer says no. It has to be signed by the UK embassy." It's enough to send you running to the nearest psychiatric hospital, where you can bounce off the walls. I nearly gave up so many times. We received the invitation for an interview two years later instead of the initially predicted: "maximum six months wait".

An official letter ordered me to present myself, accompanied by my husband, at the *préfecture* at a specific time and date. No alternative was permitted. I was given a leaflet to revise and told to be well prepared. Any evidence of a false marriage would be dealt with severely. I was starting to get a bit scared… I'd watched Gérard Depardieu get kicked out of America in the film *Green Card*.

D-day came, and we arrived, a little twitchy, dossier in hand, smartly dressed and way ahead of schedule. I could sing *La Marseillaise* off by heart, name the last five presidents and knew about naughty Napoleon and *all* the Louis. I could tell you the approximate population of the main cities and name the major rivers and mountain ranges of France on a map. I was ready. Or so I thought…

A lady who couldn't have been more than twenty-five years old called my name and led us down a corridor. Christophe was instructed to go into room No.1, and I was taken into room No.2. My stress levels were in overdrive. I gave a last helpless glance at my husband as they closed the doors.

We were to be interrogated using the same questions, to which the answers would be compared. This was in order to verify that we had not entered into a *marriage blanc* (arranged marriage). Ridiculous but apparently necessary.

"First question," the woman said. "How did you meet your 'usband?"

Flipping heck, I hadn't anticipated that. I had two options: either lie, saying we'd exchanged shy glances during a pottery class. Or tell the truth and suffer the shameful consequences. As I hadn't discussed a possible alibi with Christophe, I went with Plan B. Try and explain Hogs and Heifers to a dowdy, young French *fonctionnaire*. Her eyes and mouth opened wider and wider as I explained dancing on the bar, taking off my bra and pretending to be married, digging myself deeper and deeper into a pit.

She looked at her computer and started tapping furiously. Changing the subject abruptly, she then asked where our children went to school, what Christophe's hobbies were, and what did I like most about France? That was easy – the wine, of course!

Christophe was then ushered in for phase two.

"Just *you* answer please now, madame. What are the values of *La République?*"

Hmmm… I knew there were three. "*Liberté, Égalité* and…" Shit. My mind went totally blank.

I started to blub like a baby. Christophe kicked me under the table in his usual gallant way.

"Give me a chance! I know the answer, madame, I know the answer…" What *was* it?

"*Fraternité!*" I yelled in triumph as she nearly fell off her chair.

"*Oui.* Yes. But… what else?" *Else*? What the hell was she fishing for?

"Democracy?" That must be it. I sat back in the chair with my arms folded, feeling very pleased with myself.

"Madame Lesage." She looked me straight in the eye. "What about laicity?"

"Oh yes. Laicity. I was about to say that too."

She played her trump card. "And… what is the definition of *laicité*, may I ask?"

Pants. No idea. Something to do with religions all being equal?

"No, madame. It is the separation of the church and the state. The law was passed in 1905. *Merci.* You can go now."

Not even one question about Napoleon. I looked out of the car window miserably, sulking all the way home.

Ploughing back into my work, I started to make some amazing acquaintances. Once or twice in a lifetime, you may meet someone so incredible, so influential, and so inspirational that they completely change your whole outlook on the world and your sense of perspective, as well as your personal and professional ambitions. In my case, this person came in the form of Dr François Barbotin-Larrieu. When I grow up, I want to be just like him.

He told me his story. François worked as an anaesthetist but was also one of the leading figures of *Médecins Sans Frontières* (Doctors Without Borders) as well as being a member of an association helping underprivileged Vietnamese children receive lifesaving thoracic surgery.

He spent his summer holidays working in rural Vietnam rather than tanning himself in Bonifacio like most French doctors did. Apart from doing extremely well academically at school, he was a football ace. When François was eighteen, he'd had a choice: medical school or a place in the junior Paris Saint-Germain team. Luckily for the world, he chose medicine.

"Another great header from Barbotin-Larrieu!" Just doesn't sound right.

He was always charging off to whichever place had just suffered a natural catastrophe or started a tragic new war. Grabbing a bulletproof vest on the way out, he'd wave, "I've found a locum replacement, Kate. See you in a few days, weeks, maybe months. We'll see."

He was always discreet, dignified and extremely humble about it all. The only time I heard him brag was after meeting Angelina Jolie.

"What was she like?" I asked, in starstruck awe.

"*Son visage,* her face…" he answered wistfully, looking somewhere faraway into the distance with a sigh. "A sight to behold. *Une poésie.* A poem."

He had witnessed such horror and suffering, the likes of which most of us couldn't even begin to imagine. I bullied and cajoled information from him about his exploits out of pure fascination. We spent hours discussing the Israeli-Palestine situation.

But the one that touched me most was the story of little Landina. In 2010, a terrible earthquake hit the island of Haiti, one of the poorest places on earth. Thousands of people were killed, injured and maimed. François took the first available flight and joined a volunteer, war-zone colleague and doctor friend of his, David Nott (nicknamed Indiana in medical circles, after his daring adventures), to search for survivors amongst the rubble.

They came across the debris of a destroyed children's hospital in Port-au-Prince and noticed the tiny, fragile arm of an infant sticking out from under the stones. They looked again. *Did one of the fingers just move?* They dug her out and quickly assessed her condition. Landina had been hospitalised with severe burns a few days prior to the entire building collapsing. Most homes in Haiti didn't have electricity. They relied on candlelight. Fires were, therefore, unfortunately very common. She had been lying in agony and fear under the rubble, surrounded by dust and corpses, for at least two days.

François and David realised two things: her arm would need to be amputated in order to get her out, and specialised surgery on her crushed skull would be imperative if she was to survive. There was a surgeon at Great Ormond Street Hospital in London, willing and able to help.

The first problem was that the Haitian government had issued travel restrictions for children following a suspected child-trafficking ring. Luckily, Inigo Gilmore, a British filmmaker, was making regular reports to the media on Landina's condition. Suddenly, the whole world was talking about her: the "miracle baby". The team thus managed to obtain last-minute extradition papers to take her to the neighbouring Dominican Republic.

"We delivered her from pure hell on earth," François told me, "against all odds and unbelievable bureaucratic obstruction. Somehow, we managed to persuade them to loan us a helicopter from the embassy, and we flew across as quickly as we could. Her visa was literally handed to us on the tarmac. She was in my arms, all bandaged up but very well-behaved.

British Airways had agreed to block a flight for us to London from Punta Cana. The passengers were very understanding once they were told the reason for the delay. We made it to England just in time for the operation, which was, thank God, a total success."

Thanks to Facing the World, a British charity specialising in craniofacial reconstructive paediatric surgery, the entire medical costs were covered. Landina recovered and grew strong. She even developed a beautiful, cheeky smile despite all the trauma she'd suffered.

But had she been orphaned? Was her family looking for her? Inigo, who was also an award-winning journalist, decided to return to Haiti and find out. Searching through the rubble and wreckage, he was determined to get information on Landina, despite no helpful leads or documentation. After much probing, the surviving staff at the destroyed Trinite hospital suggested he look in a township called Bizoton. Here, he interviewed as many people as possible and met Marie Seignon, a twenty-six-year-old mother who had lost her hospitalised baby girl during the earthquake. A DNA test confirmed that she was indeed Landina's mother. She wept with joy and relief, along with Landina's three elder brothers and sisters. Ironically, the name Seignon translates into English as "miracle". Facing the World organised visas, tickets and a passport, which enabled her to spend six weeks in London, reunited with her daughter.

This tale of disaster and survival against all odds is heart-warming, indeed. But perhaps personalising tragedy is wrong.

After all, Landina eventually had to return to a country with scant access to primary healthcare, limited education facilities and a makeshift home without electricity. Not to mention the equally vulnerable population around her, all of whom did not receive the same help.

I got home that evening and sat out in our hammock under the stars. The same stars that would be above Landina just six hours later. I looked around me. I had a job, a car and a roof over my head. My children went to school, we had a family doctor consultation if needed within twenty-four hours, and three meals a day. That alone put me in the top 1% of most privileged humans on earth.

And yet the only fundamental difference between my Emilie and Landina was where they were born. One lives in a three-bedroomed house with a garden and working electricity. The other in a candle-lit room in the middle of an infested slum.

Where's the justice in that? I knew where this train of thought was going… I *had* to get over to Haiti and help.

My mind was made up even before I discussed it with Christophe. If they needed someone with my skills, I thought, I'd be willing to pay for my flight and lodgings. This would mean a huge financial sacrifice for the family; we didn't have the three thousand or so euros to spare. It would need to be begged, borrowed or stolen. The kids would just have to be put on a diet of pure pasta for a while. They'd be OK. I'd survived for years on baked potatoes.

My lovely husband was very supportive.

"Just do it," he said. "I'll work from home and look after Alex and Emilie."

Amel was very excited about the idea and agreed to give me four weeks' leave of absence. For my first humanitarian trip as a young mother, I was counting on being away for no longer than a month. MSF and the Red Cross were a no-go, their nursing expeditions are generally for much longer periods.

I contacted Adele, one of my Irish nursing friends from our crazy New York days. I knew that Kevin, her husband, made regular trips to Haiti as a volunteer doctor. Would he be able to introduce me to the right people?

Turns out, in fact, he could. And he did.

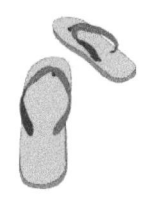

11. HAITI

One small drop in an ocean of goodwill
(and rum)

Haiti is the poorest country in the western hemisphere, on many levels. Four-fifths of the population live in absolute poverty. Seventy-five percent of Haitians live on less than two dollars a day. The minimum wage is next to nothing, three-fifths of the population are permanently unemployed and over half are illiterate.

It occupies the western third of a mountainous island in the Caribbean with stunning beaches, once a sought-after holiday destination and pirate stronghold, the Dominican Republic making up the other two-thirds. Originally, the population were almost entirely descendants of African slaves.

Haiti has a population of over eleven million, squeezed into just 28,000 km^2. It freed itself from colonial rule by the French in 1804 and then became a Republic. France demanded huge sums of money for this privilege, presumably in order to dissuade other occupied territories from doing the same. Since the split, Haiti has suffered numerous economic, social, political and natural disasters, plunging the country into chronic poverty. The 2010 earthquake and its aftershock severely damaged the capital, Port-au-Prince, and surrounding areas. An estimated 200,000 people were killed. Hundreds of thousands more were injured, and over a million became homeless.

Well-meaning peace-keeping troops arrived with the usual

non-governmental organisations. But their negligent waste disposal methods reintroduced the deadly cholera bacterium into the main river. The UN has made an official apology, but the Haitians have had to pay the bill with terrible long-term effects. Philanthropy can be disastrous, it would seem – I didn't want to go over there and make things worse. It was essential to me that I went with the *right* organisation.

Along with the earthquake, much natural vegetation has been destroyed through deforestation and population increase as townsfolk moved from Port-au-Prince into the countryside. And a lack of conservation measures has damaged animal life as well as the coral formation that protected the coastline.

Despite the potential wealth of its fertile soil, one-fifth of all food is imported, mainly from the US. Much is smuggled in, too, further impoverishing the nation's struggling farmers. Agriculture is a large part of the economy, but soil erosion, drought, and irrigation problems hinder the production of coffee, corn, yams and sugarcane.

Many try for a better life by migrating to America, Cuba or the Dominican Republic. This is often a hazardous, potentially even deadly, adventure and entire families are jammed into small rubber boats. Most people make a living doing hand-to-mouth work, selling their wares on the street and trinket-making. Illegal activities are tempting, therefore, rife.

Haitians speak *Créole* in their daily lives. It's an interesting mixture of French, German and English, with a bit of Dutch thrown in.

You are so pretty is: "*Ou tré bèl.*" I can't dance translates to "*Mwen pa konn danse.*"

French is used for more formal circumstances, but the R is replaced by a W, as in the French West Indies.

"*Il est très riche*," (he is very rich) would be pronounced, "*Il est twés wich.*"

There is no official religion in Haiti, and voodoo is widely practised. Voodoo conjures up visions of sorcery, animal sacrifices and satanic worship, but it is actually based upon ancestral spirits from the slave times and patron saints. It has become a prominent Haitian belief system, a cultural tradition and the soul of many communities. At times this is blamed for health disparities, as some say people are dissuaded from seeking conventional medical help. However, many voodoo priests in Haiti are real doctors or midwives. When working over there, it was important to respect this aspect of their culture.

Per capita, Haiti currently spends about thirteen dollars a year on healthcare, compared to one hundred and eighty dollars in the neighbouring Dominican Republic. Just one-quarter of births are medically assisted. Half the population has no direct access to healthcare due to financial barriers, and a direct payment system is in place.

Malaria, dengue, zika and chikungunya are the most common diseases. Thousands suffer from TB, HIV malnutrition, hypertension and diabetes too. Government investment in healthcare accounts for only about 4% of the state budget. The country is therefore dependent on foreign aid. As for Haiti's healthcare priorities, the World Bank is calling for a relocation of funds, with more emphasis on prevention and primary clinics. A donor culture over two generations has pushed forward photogenic projects such as shiny new hospitals, which very often fail to respond to the real needs of the country. There's a reason why Haiti is known as the "NGO Republic." But maybe the answer lies in a universal coverage system: people who can afford to will pay for health insurance, whilst people who cannot are covered by the government or private donors. A Haitian doctor earns around 15,000 pounds a year. A nurse in the region of 3,000. On a positive note, however, many world organisations recognise that the public health system in Haiti *has* progressed since the earthquake, notably through partnerships with the US under the Obama administration.

There is truth in the quotation: "You can't go back and

change the beginning, but you can start where you are and change the ending."

Kevin put me in touch with Damien, the manager of an Irish charitable foundation set up by a wealthy philanthropist, particularly engaged in helping the people of Haiti. This charity, along with many others, sponsors schools, healthcare and community work. Kevin, a renowned Dublin ophthalmologist, himself regularly intervened at the eye clinic on Île-à-Vache, an island just off the mainland.

Haitian, as well as foreign, doctors and nurses came there sporadically but didn't have the necessary experience to set up a proper working clinic. So Kevin linked up with this charity and other allies to create and fund a functioning, useful ophthalmology service.

"With the onset of menopause, a lot of Haitian women around the age of forty onwards suddenly start to lose their eyesight," he told me. "They often make jewellery and sew clothes for a living, so you can imagine the difficulties that brings. Ophthalmologic care is super important for their well-being and that of their families. There's no glory. No glamour. We just need people who are empathetic and bloody hard workers."

No need to say another word. I was in. 100%.

Having obtained my tourist and professional visas, changed some money into Haitian Gourdes, gotten a prescription for anti-malaria pills and renewed my passport, it was vaccination time. Hepatitis A, hepatitis B, typhoid, cholera, yellow fever, rabies, meningitis, polio, measles, mumps, rubella, polio, tetanus, diphtheria, pertussis, chickenpox, shingles, influenza… The list was longer than a Parisian penis extension. I looked like a used pincushion by the end of my appointment: red blotches and scabs all over my arms.

Before long, it was time to go. After much guilty kissing and cuddling at Charles de Gaulle, I abandoned Christophe and the kids and boarded my flight to Miami. The return ticket was a whole month later; I'd never been apart from them for more than a day or two before! I knew I was going to miss them all like mad.

Having said that, settling down to watch the inflight movie with a glass of prosecco in hand, a wave of excitement washed over me. This was in no small part due to the fact that I was off to a sunny Caribbean island and to be met, after the second leg of my journey, at Port-au-Prince airport by a *chauffeur* if you please.

Pushing away any glamourous assumptions I had made of a luxury limo meeting me in a palm-tree-lined paradise, *Toussaint Louverture* airport was hot and chaotic, there wasn't even a palm tree in sight. The car turned out to be a rickety old Jeep, known as a "Tap Tap" - so-called because you can only get them to stop when you tap hard on the door, twice.

The heat was like a dry, burning slap in the face. It was already hitting over 30°C at nine in the morning. Despite this, all the locals wore trousers and long-sleeved shirts; quite a few even had blazers on. I had a couple of hours to spare before I caught the boat to the Île-à-Vache, and James, the driver, asked me if I'd like to visit the town.

"Great idea!" I replied, full of touristic enthusiasm.

I was in luck; it was market day at the famous Marché de Fer.

"You'll be quite safe with me, Madame Kate," James said. "No pwoblem."

I nodded happily in agreement. I didn't feel jet lagged at all and was eager to discover this new country. James started warming to me when he realised that I was a regular, smiley person, coming here with a sincere desire to help. Not a nasty, rich *blan* – the word for white tourist. In Haiti, a smile receives a smile. I never felt targeted or at risk during my stay but rather welcomed by cheerful, friendly faces.

"Come take a look at my *beeautiful* bwacelets, chéwi!" "Good morning, pwitty lady! Coffee with a little homemade *wum* to start this lovely day?" Rum at nine-thirty in the morning! Even as a Brit, I was a little shocked. But I had one anyway.

I needed to be aware of basic safety measures and use common sense. Women alone risk being hassled, as they do in many places, unfortunately. I was told not to walk around at night, even accompanied. This was mainly to avoid being followed by people asking for money, my phone or my watch, more than anything else. Getting from A to B was always with a native driver, who was usually armed.

The Fer market was bustling, full of travellers mingling with locals. Markets are central to Haitian commerce. Colourful mosaics and paintings, wooden carvings, voodoo statues and boxes of cigars were on offer everywhere. Salsa music and drum beats played in the background, and the walls along the main streets were covered in pink and orange bougainvillea vine flowers.

This was obviously a poor town; we passed a lot of beggars, but people seemed to be happily going about their daily lives amid all the tourists. Shoe shiners, car washers and lottery ticket sellers were offering their services on every corner. Many of the city churches were still standing and busy with people walking in and out, either for worship or just a curious peek.

The traditional snack on sale everywhere was *mamba*: mini loaves of bread covered in creamy peanut butter. In between the shacks and torn-down buildings stood the Gingerbread Houses. These surviving structures are a Cuban-style architectural delight, decorated with unique latticework and ornamental carving around a timber frame, evoking a colonial fairy-tale feel.

The smell of sugar and spices wafted in the air and drew me in. Following the delicious, sweet aroma, we arrived at a small stand selling banana, rum and chilli-flavoured hot chocolate. It was divine. I had a new business plan right there. Having stimulated my taste buds, I asked James where we could go for a typical lunch. He took me down through the meandering crowds to the Latin quarter.

We stopped outside a restaurant while James talked with the hesitant guard on the door, who eventually let us in. It was basic, but the escargots and goat stew was worthy of a Michelin star. I washed it all down with a glass of very fine Viognier, knowing that my menu for the next four weeks would probably be a *lot* less gastronomic.

As we drove away from the town, heading south west, I reflected on the surprising yet authentic place that was Port-au-Prince. There was an air of rebirth in the face of destruction. Even their new president was an ex-musician known as Sweet Mickey. The people in this battered and bruised community wore hope and raw emotion on their faces, and their art, cuisine and music left me far from indifferent. In fact, it was quite the reverse – I couldn't wait to come back here on my way home.

Driving through Haiti is an incredible experience. It has a magnificent, verdant mountain range, impressive even when compared to the Alps or the Pyrenees. It looks like a mixture of Costa Rica and the Grand Canyon. Think Jurassic Park, minus the dinosaurs.

The traffic was terribly slow, like a lot of things in Haiti. Animals crossed the road without warning, blocking our path. It took hours to travel the relatively short distance. I forced myself not to fall asleep; I didn't want to miss any of the sights or scenery. Having a 4x4 vehicle wasn't a luxury, more a necessity. The road infrastructure was disastrous.

I made my boat just in time and waved goodbye to James. The boat journey (in an eight-foot wooden fishing craft) was just half an hour long, but even so, I clung on, trying not to be sick, and banished all thoughts of sharks and killer jellyfish. I concentrated on clutching onto my case and admiring the spectacular mountainous coastline, which we were gradually leaving behind.

Kevin had told me about these boats, the only transport available for the hospital ophthalmologic staff and equipment. Each piece of microscope had travelled the same way as me. He also told me that the beaches on the Île-à-Vache are amongst the most beautiful in the world. As we got closer, I realised he wasn't kidding. Check on Google Earth if you don't believe me. White sands, perfect blue skies and crystal water in every shade of green awaited me as I disembarked, a slight shade of green myself.

My new colleagues paddled barefoot over the stones and stood knee-deep in the sea to help me and my suitcase off the boat. They took me to my quarters: a charming albeit stifling hot straw hut about two hundred feet from the beach. Having dropped my stuff off, one of the aides said she'd show me around the clinic after her lunch break.

"Make yourself at home, Madame Kate. Fweshen up! Have a siesta. There's wum in the cooler. See you in an hour or two, chéwi… no hurry. *Ici, c'est Haiti*. This is Haiti." These words were to set the scene for the length of my stay.

Despite the relaxed atmosphere, I was keen and itching to get to work. Full of beans, I arrived at the clinic as scheduled. Nobody was around. We were on Haitian time. I waited for just under two hours in the shade of a palm tree sitting on the hot, itchy sand before the auxiliary nurse showed up.

"Sowwy chéwi," she said, taking a big bunch of keys out of her bag. "Siesta longer than usual. My husband, he vewy fwisky at the moment… he want another baby."

Jeepers. In her lunch break, in *this* heat?

The clinic was a box-shaped building surrounded by white bars. There were two large steps leading up to the door, upon which several locals were lounging. Half of the area was for waiting; what with the bars, it felt like a cattle shed. The other half was divided into three rooms: the nurse's station and two ophthalmology consultation suites. They were pretty well equipped – basic, but with all the necessary technology and materials.

The team were hovering around the coffee machine, having just arrived and getting ready for the afternoon shift. There were nine of us in all: four doctors, four auxiliaries and myself. They were extremely welcoming, and the simple tasks required of me were explained very clearly. Nurse volunteers came and went so often that they were well rehearsed. I spent the rest of the afternoon chatting, sweating and having a general nose-around.

Eventually, after a hearty supper of corn chilli and a sticky, sleepless night surrounded by buzzing mosquitoes, I began my Haitian voluntary project at last.

My tasks were to take the patients' obs (pulse, temperature and blood pressure) and help with the eye exams, as well as deal with any necessary blood samples. I was also expected to reorganise the off-duty, assist with the vaccination program and instigate an auxiliary nurse teaching curriculum. Managing lazy, moody Parisian youngsters was a walk in the park compared to these guys.

As Damien had told me, two generations of subservience and NGO funding, an economic calamity maketh. The other problem was the image of nursing; there was a clear demarcation – we were the doctors' handmaidens and not to be taken too seriously.

For example, after showing them how and why, I asked the auxiliaries very nicely for the instruments to be properly sterilised rather than the usual spit and polish. I was rewarded with fervent head nods, toothy smiles and, "Of cowse, chéwi. *Tout de suite*. No pwoblem." I came back three hours later, and of course, it hadn't been done.

"What's going on?" I demanded. "Why has nothing been put in the autoclave?"

Four pairs of big brown eyes stared at me.

"This is Haiti, chéwi… no stwess. Stwess not *good* for you."

I quickly learnt there are two very important things to these islanders: taking things very slowly… and sex. There's a Haitian proverb which I found summed it up well: "*Si on gade lontan ase ou ka wè bèt yo sou yon foumi.*" Which roughly translates to: If you squint long and hard enough, you can even spot tits on an ant.

At least the Wi-Fi was up to scratch, and I was able to speak regularly to Christophe and the kids via FaceTime on my new-fangled contraption known as an iPhone.

My days were spent taking care of a never-ending queue of patients; some would wait in line for five or six hours with no complaining whatsoever. We'd check their vital signs, test their vision and prescribe treatment. Most of the time they just needed glasses, but often surgery was required for cataracts, glaucoma or macular degeneration.

The problem with being on an island was that if the equipment broke down, we were basically, well… buggered. Also, any serious postoperative complications needed to be dealt with on the mainland, or a specialist had to be sailed in.

I took a keen interest in building anaesthetic protocols, teaching them which drops and products work best to make the procedures painless. The Haitian population were so used to suffering that they willingly endured eye surgery with no anaesthesia. They were unbelievably stoic and brave. There was no privacy, and there were no curtains – they just lined up in long, endless rows and waited their turn, often holding a child or two on their hips. Nobody pushed in front of anyone, and politeness reigned. But we were working fourteen to fifteen-hour days and were utterly exhausted.

In the late evening, we'd head to Smokey's Beach Bar for rum cocktails and beer. I met some incredibly devoted and interesting people, and it was an honour to hang out with them. Voluntary medical staff had come from all over, notably the UK, USA, Canada and France. Most stayed for between three and six months. Some had been working in the country for over ten years, like Damien. He was the director of this particular charitable healthcare program and a very special person.

"I went to a rural village in the mountains last week," he told me. "It was to vaccinate the babies, give family planning advice and nutritional support. These guys have nothing. And yet the tiny amount of food on offer – they gave it to me. I tried to refuse, but they *insisted*."

He took a sip of his rum and continued, "In this country, kindness is met with kindness. You show respect, and you get respected. I've never met people like them. Despite their everyday struggles we've become friends… they've even taught me to speak *Créole* and to dance! Life here is primitive, basic and tough. These people are willing to learn, work hard and take part in activities, but on the other hand, there's terrible insecurity, degrading housing and disease added to the high cost of food. Not to mention regular natural disasters… it's a matter of survival." Apparently, it all started with a bunch of pigs.

"Pigs," he explained, "were the national treasure – literally bargained with. In exchange for pig tender, you got an education for your kids, food, land, marriage ceremonies and medical care. "In the 1970s, there were over a million black pigs in Haiti until African swine flu hit the country. According to many experts, about one-third of the animals were thought to be infected. The US government, fearful of the virus reaching their shores, ordered the eradication of *all* Haitian pigs. Despite contestation, the massacre was carried out. America replaced them with stateside pink pigs, not at all adapted to the climate – they drank only fresh water, obviously not widely available. It was a disastrous idea. The economy was hit hard, further impoverishing the country but creating a boom for the US pig farming industry." He paused, looking sad, but determined.

"What this country needs is strong leadership. A government intent on upgrading farming, health, housing and schools. We can only hope that will happen one day. Here's to Haiti."

We clinked glasses and necked back our third shot of Barbancourt.

Swimming in the warm Caribbean Sea or lying on a paradisiacal beach after work was great, I admit. And I loved being woken up every morning by the sound of praying, mixed with dogs barking and cockerels crowing – a world away from my usual urban soundscape. Women came out early to arrange their wares on stalls or to start fires in preparation for cooking lunch, whilst the village children ran around barefoot, playing with anything they could get their hands on, often following me about and chattering in *Créole* or touching my hair. I was blown away by the friendliness of the people and by the beauty of the island.

But the long hours and conditions were difficult, and by the end of the month, I was seriously starting to fantasise about a proper bed, taking a bath and eating some non-spicy food. I was missing my family terribly and looking forward to returning home.

The day before I left, a visit was organised to a local orphanage; I thought I'd be heartbroken and feared I would arrive home to Christophe with at least five adopted babies. However, it was actually admirably run, and the children were taken care of superbly well. It showed me an example of where Haitians can be more than capable of managing healthcare establishments efficiently when properly directed and with their own motivated staff.

From my short experience there and after many discussions with many different people, I would agree that more delegation to preventative care and non-medical staff in order to reduce the doctors' workload is necessary. Nurses (and opticians) have enough training to handle clinics and do the IVTs (injections for macular degeneration). Centralising care with integrated services on the mainland could also be helpful, according to Damien.

Sterility, waste disposal and hygiene need to be prioritised. Simple, regular hand washing isn't yet fully instilled in Haitian culture – it's not so easy when you don't have clean running water and soap. Sexually transmitted diseases and unwanted pregnancies were also major problems for obvious reasons. Women's health needed to be addressed in a more urgent manner, I felt.

The country has some of the richest natural reserves on the planet. And yet it is crippled by poverty and chaotic administration. The untapped potential is palpable. In order to rebuild their integrity, the Haitian people need to let the healing process begin and stop the almost 100% external control. By relearning farming, tourism, medical and commercial skills, they will regain autonomy and a sense of national pride stolen from them so cruelly in the wake of the natural disasters. Not forgetting those greedy American politicians, too – let's be honest.

Mine was a brief, frustrating at times, but extremely fulfilling and humbling experience. It was a momentous privilege to have been part of this wonderful community, even for a short while. It was also uplifting to think that so many people from around the world refuse to turn a blind eye to suffering and inequality and get out there to help. The trip had somewhat restored my faith in humanity.

I knew I'd be back once the kids had grown up a bit, so the goodbyes weren't *too* painful, though a few hidden tears were shed behind my sunglasses as James drove me back to Port-au-Prince.

Arriving at Charles de Gaulle, I've never felt so much love, gratitude and happiness at seeing those three smiling faces waiting for me. I'd expected sulks, tantrums and guilt trips, but actually, they seemed proud of me and wanted to hear all about it. I felt proud of *myself* that I'd followed my dream and that my children saw their mum as a positive role model.

The situation we were thrown into days later made me feel even more resolved in this regard. The dreaded summons to the HR office at nine in the morning in a company that was restructuring could only mean one thing – Christophe, along with half of his team, was made redundant. And as anyone who's been through this knows, it's just as hard morally as it is financially. There was a lot of anger, disappointment and low self-esteem.

I started to work full-time, did extra agency shifts at the weekends to make more money and tried my best to reassure and be supportive. But those were dark times that tested our marriage and pushed us to the edge of bankruptcy. If it hadn't been for our parents' help, we would have found ourselves in rather dire straits.

On the bright side, my French nationality came through! Laicity obviously wasn't such a big deal after all. I went to work the next day acting thoroughly rude to everyone. I parked my car sideways, taking up two parking spaces. I talked loudly about my union right to strike and pushed in at the cafeteria, refusing to wait in line. I pouted, sneered and made lots of tutting and annoyed "ooh la *la!*" noises whilst looking down my nose at people.

Already a true *française*. But a second-degree one, I assure you.

They say that you are culturally integrated when you start to dream in the language of a country. I beg to differ. It's when you really start to swear like them.

I noticed that I now said *"merde"* as often as "shit." This thought stirred a proud swelling in my chest; I felt at home in this land and was starting to truly love it. Shit and *merde* were also our kids' two preferred words after having dropped food from their highchair, losing a toy or banging themselves on the head. Now *that's* bilingualism.

Then, after more than six months of searching, countless dead ends and failed interviews, Christophe sat the family down at the kitchen table one evening to tell us he'd been offered a job. We saw the old cheeky grin and sparkle back in his eyes.

"Just one minor detail," he said.

"What's that?"

"It's in London!"

Holy crap! I'd just become French for nothing.

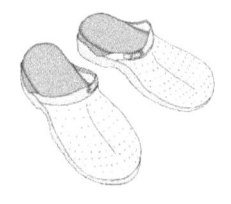

12. CAMBRIDGE

NHS Revisited

Whoever said the grass is greener was right.

After the initial euphoria, reality hit home. Shock number one was the price of renting accommodation in London. That's when I learnt about the dreadful "catchment area" phenomenon. So now only the rich or very lucky can send their kids to good schools! Causing a vicious circle promoting a two-tier system. Fair? I think *not*.

We looked at private schools (there's a French *lycée* in Kensington) and nearly choked when we saw the fees. So, after examining our options, we decided it would be best to live outside London, where it was *slightly* cheaper, and Christophe would just have to commute. It was my dad who suggested Cambridge, as he now lived and worked there. He told us that the commute to King's Cross was reasonably quick. What he omitted to mention was that, even in cattle class, fares would cost about half of Christophe's salary. A first-class monthly pass would swallow the lot.

Being used to French TGVs running smoothly along at 200 mph, Christophe found the rickety chugging of British Rail uncomfortable, crowded, horrifically expensive, as I said, and often unfashionably late. It was a bit of a culture shock.

"Thatcher's government bought all the railway infrastructure, but the operators charge what the hell they want, benefitting from huge subsidies, so the commuters end up paying twice. It's the biggest taxpayer looting scam in the history of Britain!"

He wasn't exactly what you might call a big B.R. fan.

We found a lovely, large, converted barn to rent on the outskirts of Cambridge. There were a couple of nice local pubs and a supposedly "outstanding" village primary school. As schooling in the UK is compulsory, I foolishly imagined that our kids would be admitted to the local public one automatically and soon be running off in their uniforms, clutching satchels, packed lunches and conkers on strings. What we found, however, was that there were no places available. The council gave us two choices: send them to a school with a very dodgy reputation twenty miles away or teach them from home. I decided on the latter and made the necessary inscriptions to the online international distance learning organisation – the CNED.

The coursework was tedious and boring. I had to be constantly behind them with my whip and megaphone, ensuring the homework was handed in on time. And, of course, there was zero interaction with other students, which wasn't helping their English. I half expected the police or social services to come knocking, but nobody ever checked on their progress or showed the slightest bit of concern that they weren't at school. I made the daily trip on the bus to the local education authority building, demanding an update on waiting list places. I think in the end they got so fed up with me (people would hide under their desks when I walked in) that they eventually decided to simply increase the class capacities.

Like Pinocchio then, Alex and Emilie finally got to be *real* children, wear a uniform and trot off to school every morning. It had only taken five flipping months. School was tricky in the beginning. Bullying reared its ugly head. There were tears and tantrums and cries of, "*On ne comprend rien!*" We don't understand anything! But little by little, their English improved to an astonishing level. They were even in the end-of-term school plays. Looking back, despite everything, we agree it was the best thing we have ever done for our kids.

Now that I wasn't home-schooling, I started to look for employment. We needed money to buy train tickets. A piece of cake, I said to myself. Nurses were in demand as they were everywhere, and I'd kept up my registration to the UK NMC (Nursing and Midwifery Council).

I made photocopies of my diplomas, typed out a CV in English and headed confidently off to the local hospital, which was advertising for an *anaesthetic assistant*. I'd tried applying online, using the NHS website, but having had an unusual professional career path, the computer hadn't understood. So, I decided to just pop along.

The head theatre nurse who met with me was a very nice man and organised an interview with the anaesthetic medical staff. I regurgitated all the correct answers to the usual questions, smiled politely and agreed enthusiastically to perform menial tasks for a pittance. The job required little experience, no formal qualifications and would hold practically zero responsibility. I'd have done it happily just to get out of the house.

They turned me down, arguing that I had a French diploma which wasn't valid in the UK. This wasn't strictly true, I protested, and I also had a valid English one – I'd given them a copy! Plus, neither was necessary, according to the job description.

I wrote to the hospital administrator to ask for an honest explanation, but they never found the time to reply. When I called back, the head nurse nervously explained in an apologetic tone that the doctors weren't happy about hiring a *nurse* who seemed to know as much as them. I'll never know if that's true, but I do hope it wasn't.

If this is what trying to find NHS hospital employment is like, I thought to myself, I'd be better off doing agency work.

Nursing agencies hire temporary replacements for people on sick leave, maternity leave or for positions that nobody else wants, mostly in old people's nursing homes. I was sent to many.

I've always adored looking after the elderly, but there have to be good conditions, healthy food, group activities and adequate staffing levels. Getting to know the residents is vital to fully supporting them medically and emotionally. Each person has specific needs, so a multidisciplinary approach is critical, and it's a far from easy job for all involved.

Fixed costs are high. Many care-home owners become extremely wealthy by cutting them in order to avoid impacting profitability. Some of the care I witnessed bordered on the abuse Estelle had described simply as a result of understaffing. These care-home shareholders obviously don't imagine that it may be *them* one day, lying in wet sheets: hungry, thirsty, cold and covered in bed sores. The unthinkable becomes routine. The routine becomes normal. Then before you know it, normal becomes acceptable. Treating old people like this is *not* acceptable.

The population was ageing fast (as it continues to do), and already 450,000 elderly people in the UK lived in long-term care homes, costing on average eight hundred pounds per week; way more than most retirement budgets allow. Governments worldwide, not just in the UK, need to invest massively in these essential infrastructures.

Despite the bliss of being able to see Jo, Julia and all the other people I'd missed on a more regular basis – not to mention prawn cocktail crisps, Marmite sandwiches and sticky toffee pudding – I was a little disappointed with certain other altered aspects of my beloved country.

For a start, there seemed to have been an invasion of Big Brother. Cameras called CCTV were everywhere. Literally. You couldn't pick your nose discreetly at the bus stop any more without being filmed.

Speaking of buses, on which I'd spent a large chunk of my childhood, we'd always been taught to give up our seats for someone more in need. Now, it seemed, public transport was populated by indifferent zombies, headphones stuck to their ears, eyes fixed on the floor. The elderly and physically impaired could damn well stand up. Or try to anyway. I began to realise that coming back to England for the weekend was rosier than actually living there full-time. Unless you've got tons of money.

Cambridge is a truly beautiful place, though, and undoubtedly one of the most impressive cities in England. We ambled around the city centre market amongst the students and tourists, trying to avoid being run over by thousands of bicycles whilst admiring the magnificent towering Gothic chapel of King's College. The spectacular fan vaulting inside of which is sometimes considered to be one of the wonders of the world.

Famous for its prestigious, ancient university, Cambridge is situated in the east of England, surrounded by flat fenlands. The thirty-one university colleges make up about a third of all buildings in the old town. Wandering around, you could be forgiven for thinking you've gone back a couple of centuries. There are winding, picturesque riverside walks, olde worlde inns with beamed ceilings selling draught ale, and the historic market, which bustles with energy, local culture and noise. There are narrow cobblestone roads and alleyways leading to pubs, quaint little parks and numerous coffee shops selling cream buns and aromatic hot chocolate, all sprinkled with hundreds and thousands. Our favourite pub was The Eagle, the city's oldest one, decorated in graffiti by American WW2 officers.

We weren't allowed access everywhere, however. Many parts were, and still are, "Professors and students only". There's a feeling of a forbidden city within a city, the great divide between *town* and *gown*.

During the famous, lavish May Ball season, young students roam around in black tuxedos and sumptuous evening dresses, swigging from bottles of Bollinger. This marks the end of the academic year and it's serious party time.

RAG week, which begins in September, has been a seven-day-long tradition at Cambridge for over a hundred years. The students come back after summer vacation and embark on university-run charitable fundraising events, often involving large amounts of alcohol. In recent years, they seem to have calmed down a bit. A few of the naughtier antics have included climbing up the highest chapel spires to place traffic cones for all to see, hoisting a car onto the Senate roof, hijacking police vehicles and generally running around the place, either in fancy dress or naked. Nowadays, they raise thousands of pounds for charity using slightly more subtle behaviour.

If you want to see sublime caramel-coloured architecture, breath-taking bridges, impressive monuments, and picnic whilst punting down a beautiful river, go to Cambridge. Not Oxford. As anyone in Cambridge will tell you: it's *much* nicer.

The agency started sending me to work at the big teaching hospital, Addenbrooke's. They had a modern gynaecology and obstetrics wing, in which I helped run the breast clinic with a fabulous team. I worked on intensive care, the diabetic unit, theatre recovery and the outpatients' department, as well as a little stint on the medical and surgical wards before coming back to my first love: A & E.

There is a saying for women who have their babies by elective caesarean section as being "too posh to push". In the snooty Cambridge Accident and Emergency department, the clientele was obviously too posh to push… *stuff up their backsides*. I saw nothing of that whatsoever. *I don't think we're in Brighton any more, Toto.* Shoving sharp objects down their urethras, however, seemed to be fashionable amongst the gentlemen townsfolk. Knitting needles, chopsticks… even an iPhone charger. Ouch! It kept the urology house officers busy anyway, one of whom I had lunch with one day at the staff cafeteria.

She was complaining about all of the IT bureaucratic work that doctors now had to do. It was the era of computerising medical dossiers and nursing tasks, and I had to learn new keyboard skills too. Wi-Fi had started to emerge in French hospitals around the time we left Paris, and I noticed that doctors and nurses were spending more time staring into screens than looking at the patients. This, I felt, was the direct result of everything becoming digitalised – and it was something I struggled with.

The young urology doctor told me a story from her recent medical school days. She was on a ward round with a bunch of other juniors, following the great, god-like consultant around from patient to patient like ducklings waddling behind their mother. They came to Mrs Davis's bed. She had been admitted with acute pancreatitis. The consultant asked lots of questions about this particularly complex pathology, trying to destabilise and embarrass as many of the students as possible for his own amusement.

During twenty red-faced minutes, they peered together at the notes on the computer, analysing the day's rather alarming blood results. After adjusting her medication accordingly, it was time to examine the X-rays, ultrasounds and PET scans. The students were asked one by one to interpret what they thought they saw. Interestingly, nobody saw the same thing.

About twenty-five minutes after arriving at the foot of her bed, the group all turned to actually look at the patient. Mrs Davis was as dead as a dodo. No one had even noticed.

An enormous change had taken place in the nursing profession during my absence from the UK: Project 2000. Implemented in 1990, it was a scheme to change higher education, whereby nurses would attend British universities rather than nursing schools, replacing the former apprenticeship system. This meant that nursing had become a profession rather than a vocation. Nursing students were now supernumerary. Academic studies replaced hands-on care on the wards. And this all happened without an associated pay rise or improved general consideration.

The results were predictably awful. Suddenly the health service had to survive without the students' help. A higher workload for qualified nurses with added stress led to a new phenomenon called "burnout" and a massive staff turnover.

Because of this, junior, inexperienced staff were quickly promoted to senior roles. The university curriculum did not include as wide a range of specialities as it did in our day, which meant that it was hard for student nurses to choose their preferred area of work. Many newly qualified nurses headed straight for GP practices, agency work or the private sector, where the pay was simply higher than in the NHS.

There is a real risk that one day soon, there may not *be* any more qualified nurses. When we trained, we received super cheap accommodation and a small salary. Now a nursing course costs nine thousand pounds per year, just like any other degree. Except that, most other degrees will lead to decently paid employment without the stress of daily life-and-death situations in an overburdened health service. So where is the incentive for people to take up nursing? Why not do something else, something easier and better paid instead?

The other gigantic balls-up the government made was to privatise hospital porter and cleaning services. In the 1980s, our wonderful porters knew all our names, came to all the parties and worked their butts off as part of the dedicated team, starting early and finishing late if need be. Porters transfer patients, supplies, medical equipment and samples between different hospital departments and services. The cleaning staff were also vigilant, devoted and thorough. No hospital could function without them.

I remember one of them, Aaliyah, saying to me, "Kate, love! Come and look at little Junior in room twelve. He's a bit pale today, don't you think?"

Junior, who was six and had been admitted for a heart arrhythmia, was of African descent, as was our charming cleaning lady. I couldn't tell if he was pale, but she obviously could. We checked his red blood cell count again; she was right. It had gone down. He was becoming severely anaemic from an invisible cardiac bleed (hemopericardium), the causes of which can be tuberculosis, certain cancers and trauma. Aaliyah had possibly saved his life.

Nowadays, we have bugs like MRSA instead. The cleaning staff used to be attributed to one ward and knew the place off by heart. Devoted to the patients and vigorous in their work, they kept those bugs at bay.

Now, I adore the NHS. It's a national treasure, an institution in which we should all take great pride. I admire those who work in it enormously. I was born in an NHS hospital. I'll possibly die in one. The NHS trained me and gave me my chance to work in a profession that I love in many ways. There's so much great work being done in it. But, like with all big machines, parts can malfunction. The politicians in charge, as well as the general public, need to be aware of this in order to demand proper services and make changes for the better.

For the first time in forty years, UK junior doctors were going on strike from routine, and even some emergency, duties. NHS employers, acting on a government initiative, wanted to negotiate new contracts that removed a large chunk of overtime pay. These young physicians work massively long hours (people are sick day and night, and the majority of patients are seen initially by the lowly, exhausted house officer). The BMA, British Medical Association, and its unions argued that this would lead to an overall pay cut of around 40%.

Imagine 40% less salary every month. Doctors, like nurses, should be getting pay *increases,* not the opposite!

Not wishing to encourage a blame culture, there are still many frustratingly sad yet empowering stories that need to be shared to help people truly understand what it is like to be a patient or their loved one. Talking about the bad, as well as the good stuff, is the only way to increase awareness and fight against malpractice without targeting individuals. Untold stories need to be heard.

The one closest to my heart involves my dear friend Julia and her father-in-law, Peter.

Peter would have been seventy as I write this. He was entering into a well-deserved retirement in his dream cottage in the Peak District that he'd completely refurbished with his wife. Born in Lancashire into a working-class family, he'd worked extremely hard his whole life, helping to raise his own large family, with whom he was besotted. He was terribly proud of his eldest son becoming a policeman, then a senior inspector at Scotland Yard. He adored Julia and escorted her down the aisle at their wedding, her own dad being deceased. Like his son, he had a great sense of humour and loved a good gossip over a pint.

He was in terrific shape, cycling everywhere and playing golf at weekends. The only health issue he had was a minor form of irritable bowel syndrome. This is a relatively common, long-term disorder affecting the large intestine. The symptoms are constipation, gas, bloating and liquid stools. It's annoying and embarrassing but rarely dangerous unless dehydration results from prolonged symptoms – which is what happened to Peter.

He went to his GP one day, not feeling very well. He'd been having regular bouts of diarrhoea for about a week. His blood pressure was low, and his blood creatinine level was elevated (a sign that his kidneys were not working properly). His GP suggested he go to the local Accident and Emergency room for rehydration and wrote a referral.

As usual, A&E was saturated, and he wasn't seen until late that evening. They eventually did a blood test and found that his electrolytes were, predictably, totally out of whack. Our bodies are complex, intricate, delicate machines, the slightest imbalance of which can deregulate them. This body balance is called homeostasis, and when it is no longer maintained, life-threatening conditions can occur.

We have very specific levels of electrolytes in our system (potassium, calcium, magnesium, sodium and chlorine, for example). These are kept at certain levels with the help of our kidneys. When we are severely dehydrated with diarrhoea, for instance, we lose water and electrolytes, our blood pressure can drop, and our kidneys may start to suffer.

Over 60% of the human body is made up of water, and if we allow it to become dehydrated, major organs in the body can become injured. The state of dehydration occurs when water intake is less than water loss. Signs of this are muscle cramps, palpitations, light-headedness, weakness, nausea, decreased urine output (or dark urine) and a dry mouth and skin. Eventually, organ failure, coma and death may occur if untreated. In Peter's case, water and electrolytes were coming out… and so needed to be put back in. It's really not rocket science.

Unbelievably, nobody thought to put an IV catheter in Peter. They stuck a nasogastric tube down his nose into his stomach in case he went into intestinal occlusion. They gave him sips of water to drink. But the water in his stomach obviously just came straight back up out of the nasal tube…

He only saw a doctor for a few minutes, and then it was the service's healthcare assistants who popped by from time to time, peering behind the curtains to see how he was. As soon as Julia finished work – as a high-ranking practice nurse manager – she raced over to be with him. Her expert eyes immediately realised that the lifesaving drip hadn't been put in, and she went to find a nurse.

"We'll be there in a minute," she was told. They stayed the whole night in the A&E cubicle, and still no IV. The only person in the place who'd passed their mandatory IV cannula insertion certificate was the anaesthetist, who was busy in the operating room.

Of course, some of the nurses knew very well how to put one in, but doing it without the proper certificate apparently meant you get thrown into a pit of flesh-eating crocodiles and burnt in hell for eternity or some similar nonsense. In any case, it's forbidden.

Julia started losing her temper, quite rightly. She was about to put the IV in herself. Peter was starting to show signs of severe dehydration: difficulty breathing, fast heart rate, dizziness and confusion. His skin was paper dry, and his eyeballs sunken… yet *still* no IV.

Julia phoned the on-call A+E doctor again and again, told him who she was and pleaded with him to come and examine Peter. He dismissed her rudely, as silly people with power and a grudge tend to do.

"Don't tell me how to do my job!" she was told. "You're only a nurse."

Eventually, the morning shift sister came and put fluids up. At last! The only hiccup was that it wasn't fixed correctly and came out of the vein into the surrounding tissues. You can tell when this happens as the hand or arm starts to swell and become painful.

When Julia called to get someone to come and put another IV in, you can imagine the reaction she got. Unfortunately, this cost poor Peter another day of suffering. He didn't know where he was any more and kept shouting, which made the family even more unpopular with the staff.

After three days in the emergency room, he was moved to a ward, and a drip was put in and fixed securely. The problem was that his kidneys had now been irreversibly damaged. He'd also suffered a fall whilst trying to get out of bed to find some water and had hit his head. Nobody had thought to put the bedside barriers up, which is just basic nursing care. The patient next to him witnessed it all. "He kept on and on pressing the buzzer, saying he really needed to drink something… but nobody came. In the end, he tried to go it alone. I heard his head crack loudly on the floor, and I started to yell for help."

To top it all off, he now had a urinary tract infection: one of the results of a nearly empty bladder and concentrated urine. This exacerbates confusion. Peter's condition really started to deteriorate. He was slipping in and out of consciousness and having seizures. The family were beside themselves with worry.

"I immediately suspected a subdural hematoma (brain bleed) from the fall," Julia told me. "He needed to be in intensive care with a central line, a noradrenaline perfusion and intracranial pressure monitoring. They came round to do an ECG on him, but there was no paper in the machine. Nobody knew how to put the paper in, Kate. So I did it. Can you imagine such incompetence?" She started to weep at the memory.

I hugged her and listened, as would anyone. But once again, their cries for help fell on deaf ears, and he stayed on the ward for another whole day. Then, by pure luck, one of the hospital dietitians was visiting the patient in the next bed and knew Julia's family.

"Oh my God, is that *Peter*?" she exclaimed, horrified.

Immediately, she put out a cardiac arrest call; this is a special number that each hospital has, which simultaneously beeps the on-call anaesthetist, A&E senior registrar, the cardiac unit sister and her/his team to take charge of emergency situations. They have about a minute to get to the scene.

Within half an hour, Peter was properly taken care of: he was intubated, had a central line (an IV directly into the body's larger veins) and urinary catheter put in and was whisked up to ICU. But his luck was running out.

Firstly, it was a medical student who put in the intracranial monitoring line. Looking at the hospital notes years later, the reading was permanently on zero: pretty much impossible and totally abnormal. The normal value is between 10 and 15mmHg. It was very probably incorrectly positioned.

Secondly, it was the auxiliary care workers who filled out his fluid chart (what goes in and what comes out). This should be specific to the millilitre. After he had been extubated, for example, "…had some sips H_2O…" and "…used the urinal…" was written on the care chart. Not exactly precise measurements.

Nobody was treating his urine infection, either. His skin was turning mottled, which is an indication of gravity. He needed antibiotics, but they weren't given "…because he doesn't have a temperature anymore." No shit, Sherlock. That's because he was in end-stage sepsis and heading towards shock… and death. His body no longer had the energy to attack bacteria.

The nail in his coffin was that, unbelievably, the ICU sister made it clear that they needed his bed for a new admission. As he had been extubated, they said he could go to the step-down unit. "He's talking normally now, so he'll be fine," one of the nurses told them.

Julia discretely filmed Peter; he was mumbling incoherently, almost unconscious. She used this film in her legal battle later on. "I told them it would be his death sentence to move him off ICU," Julia said. "But they moved him, anyway… calling me a right pain in the arse under their breath."

Peter died about two hours later from multi-organ failure.

For every case like this, there are thousands of patients saved or well cared for in the NHS. But the moral of the story is that the NHS needs to listen to patients' families. They know the patient better than anyone.

"All we wanted was someone to hear us," said Peter's widow. "They didn't like that Julia knew her stuff. Their egos were threatened – that was more important than my husband's life."

When examining a patient, there are paraclinical signs (blood pressure, oxygen saturation, ICP intracranial pressure) which are readings on a monitor interpreted by computers. But more importantly, there are clinical signs: skin turgor, colour, breathing, sweating and consciousness levels. These, along with observations by folk who know the person well, will always tell you more about the state of a patient's health than a machine.

As a professional, Julia has had a hard time accepting what happened. "The family couldn't find peace. We needed to hear that someone was sorry. And that it would never happen again."

They consulted a lawyer and decided to instigate a malpractice suit via the NHS Ombudsman; they weren't looking for money, they wanted apologies. And change.

Doctors, and nurses for that matter, are not always right about care issues. You are allowed to – respectfully – disagree. Think of your healthcare as a partnership; it's not one-sided. And if you want to consult your notes, medical providers in the UK have thirty days in which to provide you with copies.

When Julia read Peter's records, it became overwhelmingly obvious that huge mistakes had been made concerning his care. The basic fluid input/output chart should show a balance of zero. Like the books in an accountant's office. Peter's balance was *minus ten litres*. An adult's total blood volume is normally only five litres. They literally dried him to death. Like a raisin out in the sun.

At around the same time, "The Cavendish Review" came out. Substandard care in two Staffordshire hospitals had come to light. The estimation was that between 2005 and 2009 around 1,200 people lost their lives needlessly. The neglect was appalling, scandalous and unforgivable.

The review of what went wrong suggests cover-ups by managers who attempted to cut costs in order to achieve the coveted "Foundation" status. Staff who disobeyed were threatened with the sack and feared prosecution. The government had installed a maximum four-hour waiting time in A&E: impossible to achieve unless you double staffing levels. Or falsify records.

Maybe these politicians could come and help out at the hospital sometime... it would be interesting to see how they'd cope. Over the course of eighteen months, one local family lost four members, including a baby. A nationally renowned place of safety had become a danger zone. And quite rightly, victims started wanting to see the people responsible held accountable.

The legal process took Peter's family over three years to get to a hearing. Julia represented them and did an incredible job studying the case, collecting evidence and standing up in court against powerful lawyers and consultants. She had an answer to every argument and counter-attacked like a pro. Her professional knowledge, energy, determination, and love for her father-in-law shone through.

The judge ruled in her favour. It was a huge defeat for the NHS; they were ordered to make immediate changes to the system, notably concerning the role of healthcare assistants.

It just goes to show that anybody can go up against the system and win. Whilst the family never did get a formal apology, the hospital admitted misconduct, meaning that closure was possible, at last.

The straw that broke our particular camel's back was a health problem closer to home. Christophe came back from a business trip in San Francisco, and I picked him up at Heathrow. He was exhausted and hadn't been looking after himself, notably not drinking enough water. He had severe, sharp right-side and back pain which came in waves and he had blood in his urine. You didn't have to be Einstein to work out that it was probably a kidney stone.

Trying to get to see a doctor on a Sunday afternoon in London was proving more difficult than an audience with the Queen. It wasn't *quite* bad enough to go to the hospital, according to the 999 spokesperson, so eventually, we found a small walk-in clinic on the northeast city outskirts which was open.

An obviously overworked, fed-up, but kind Indian doctor ushered us in. She prescribed painkillers and "wide spectrum" antibiotics, sure that it was an infection, but without testing the urine for specific germs; this is normally done to make sure that the right antibiotic "family" is used.

Things just got worse and worse. He couldn't sleep or work, and he was rolling around in agony. We called our GP on Monday morning. It took nineteen tries before we got through. We were told that there wouldn't be a place available till Wednesday. At the earliest.

"My company has private healthcare insurance," Christophe remembered. "Eureka!"

We called them up; at last we could cash in on those huge monthly payments. After handing over his credit card details, Christophe explained his symptoms to a curious secretary and asked to make an immediate appointment.

"Have you ever had anything remotely resembling this before?"

"Well," Christophe explained, "some years ago, I had a slight urine infection… but it was nothing like this."

"That's called a *pre-existing* condition," she replied. "So it's not covered by insurance. We can't treat you unless you pay the full costs in advance."

We looked at each other in astonishment. "I'll book the Eurostar," I said. We travelled to Paris and he got treated that same day. Hey presto!

Returning back to London two days later, minus a couple of kidney stones, we talked about it and realised that it was time to face facts; we simply didn't have the wealth to survive in modern-day southern England.

The secondary schools which the kids were destined for had terrible OFSTED (the U.K education standards office) ratings as well as drug and knife crime issues. Private schooling was out of the question at twenty-five grand a year (*per child*) Health problems… forget it. I couldn't find a permanent job, even at a lowly grade, and Christophe was exhausted from commuting. We were overdrawn to the max and surviving on beans and potatoes, like back in my student days. Income tax was the highest in Europe, yet we couldn't work out what it was being spent on. Certainly not upgrading trains, schools or hospitals.

Our England dream had turned into a disastrous, nightmarish farce. Christophe was starting to regret the whole thing. But, as always, a phone call arrived just in the nick of time. A head-hunter was interested in offering Christophe a job in Geneva. Would he consider it?

"Switzerland?" I said haughtily. "No way! Too bloody posh and boring for me."

Christophe showed me the salary proposal. I bounded up the stairs two at a time to pack our suitcases.

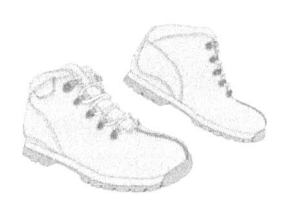

13. GENEVA

Eyes and lows

Perhaps, when you think about Switzerland, cuckoo clocks, crooked bankers, expensive watches and lederhosen spring to mind. That's what I used to believe, anyway. So it was a very nice surprise to find that Geneva (*not* the capital city, that's Bern, by the way) actually has quite an exciting, modern and vibrant buzz about it.

Situated at the westernmost point of Switzerland (which shares its border with France, Italy, Germany, Austria and tiny Liechtenstein) and surrounded by high peaks, including the majestic Mont Blanc, Geneva is nestled on the shores of the crystal-blue Lac Léman (Lake Geneva) – the largest lake in Western Europe.

It is the earth's hub for NGOs (non-government organisations), the United Nations, diplomatic organisations and, of course, banking. The Swiss are fiercely neutral and tolerant, promoting free trade and independence. They are also incredibly competitive, efficient and open-minded. Their political system is federal-based and decentralised; authority is dispersed by each district or *canton*. This gives power to local officials, and the Swiss are extremely proud of this, always turning out to vote in high numbers.

Geneva is still one of the most expensive cities in the world in which to live, almost no one can afford to buy a house or even an apartment there. However, poverty lies at 8%, wages are competitive in order to compensate for the high living costs, and the unemployment rate is at around 4%. Income tax is relatively low and taken directly out of one's wages. There is also a very generous childcare allowance available to all.

The financially intelligent (if not a little sneaky) thing to do, is live in a neighbouring cheaper country such as France and go to work every day across the border – which is exactly what we opted for. We became *frontaliers*… the equivalent of crossing over from Mexico to the US every morning. Only with slightly less risk of being cavity-searched. We easily found a house to rent, not far from the Swiss *douane,* the customs checkpoint or "rectal examination post", as Christophe poetically put it.

This best-of-both-worlds, seemingly ideal scenario needs to be weighed up, though, because it doesn't come for free. First, you have to find a job and get your Right to Practice which comes with a hefty fee. Then, apply for a work visa and qualify for a special G permit. Nurses also need to apply to the Swiss Red Cross in order to get their certificates validated. Again, not cheap. Or quick.

Passing the border every morning and evening in rush-hour traffic requires the patience of a saint, a reliable car and paying high motorway toll fees. Not to mention suffering that alarm clock beeping annoyingly at about 5.00 a.m.

Christophe, then I, discovered that constantly changing bureaucratic rules exist there and, more worryingly, there was no real ethical work code, either; people were fired without warning and sometimes for no obvious reason. Despite all this, I quite fancied nursing in yet another new country. I scoured the internet for job offers and replied to one looking for an anaesthetic nurse to join their team at a small clinic in a district of Geneva called Carouge.

They specialised in ophthalmology. This was considered the lowliest of all surgeries for an anaesthetist, there being little need for adrenaline pumps, invasive monitoring or blood transfusions.

This snobbery was misplaced, as I had already witnessed in

Haiti. I was to discover further what a great speciality eye surgery actually is. The patients, being mostly quite elderly, present multiple pathologies. The caring, communicative side of our profession is an absolute necessity. People of *all* ages are terrified at the idea of someone sticking a surgical knife or needle in their eye. Understandably so! If it was me, I'd probably bolt for the door… or just pass out.

Reassurance and gentleness were the order of the day, then. It is also incredibly fulfilling and important to help somebody to see better. Most of us would rather lose a leg than an eye, after all.

Still, there's no gore or blood and often not even any need for anaesthesia. Usually, it's the doctors and nurses nearing retirement who take this sort of position. But the team was really nice, the place spanking new, there were no on-calls or weekends, and the salary they offered seemed generous – I signed on the dotted line.

In a city of around 200,000 people, 45% of Geneva's population, like Grenoble's, is made up of ex-pats. There are, therefore, a vast number of international schooling options to choose from, both in and around the city. Not being able to afford the huge private fees, we enrolled our kids in the local French state school. It didn't have a fantastic reputation, but it was still light years ahead of what we'd experienced in Cambridge's public secondary school system. *And* they had places available.

It was an enormous relief to settle so quickly after our last hellish experience, and reminded me of a Craig David song with a few alterations:

Got a house on Monday.
Kids were in school on Tuesday.
Found a job by Wednesday.
Moved Thursday, Friday and Saturday.
We chilled on Sunday.

We explored Geneva and its surrounding areas. I loved hearing the multitude of languages as I went about my daily routines. There are ultra-cosmopolitan, bohemian districts full of heaving bars, cafés and restaurants. The old medieval town is the heart of Geneva, with its churches, squares and art galleries. Chocolate is everywhere. I think I once heard a British comedian say that this was to sweeten the Swiss image, conveniently making everyone forget about all the stolen Nazi gold. The business and shopping district is close to the lake, where locals, tourists and students lazed around on the grass in the Jardins Anglais or queued up for a boat ride on one of the Louisiana-style paddle wheel boats. We watched the world's tallest fountain shoot water 140 metres into the air from a jetty, visible for miles around.

Flea market stallholders and artists set up stands on the maze of cobbled streets which wind alongside the Rhône. I window-shopped some of the most expensive clothes and jewellery stores on the planet, then wandered around the famous vintage clothing, chocolate and watchmaker shops. You could, if you wanted to, of course, find a place to stash and clean your ambiguously-earned cash. People come to Geneva for other reasons than Toblerone.

There are heaps of wonderful museums, a beautiful public outdoor pool, a sailing club and, on a sunny day, you can rent a bicycle and travel around the hillside vineyards, or take the cable car up the Salève mountain from where you can almost see to the end of the lake.

We visited the glorious, nearby flowery town of Chamonix (don't pronounce the X, or they'll make fun of you; it's how the locals spot foreigners) nestled at the base of the most dramatic – and highest – of all European peaks: Mont Blanc. We took the little red train to the Mer de Glace, which shows unequivocally the alarming rate of global warming.

This place is also a hiker's dream, and we made the six-kilometre trek to the spectacular Lac Blanc (White Lake) via a *télécabine*. We spotted marmottes old and young alike, and paused at a refuge for a welcome ice cream – which stopped the kids whinging about their sore feet for about five seconds – while breathing in the crisp, fresh mountain air, contemplating life and feeling incredibly lucky to have landed in such beautiful surroundings.

Switzerland's healthcare system is known to be amongst, if not *the* very best. It is regulated by the federal government and is universal. Basic private insurance is obligatory, however, and certain other costs are covered by a franchise deducted annually, ranging from three hundred to four hundred Swiss francs per person per month, depending on their income and age. Ten per cent of excess costs are met by the individual, encouraging public responsibility.

Insurance companies are obliged to offer their services everywhere in the country to everyone, whatever their health status, for the same price, thus avoiding double standards and, in theory, unethical practice.

Healthcare during pregnancy is free; however, some specialities, such as dentistry, require a second coverage. The cost is, therefore, high, but then so are Swiss wages. Plus, all health services are generally rapidly available and of top quality.

For a nurse, the Swiss healthcare worker hierarchy is extremely authoritarian. The doctor is the boss and is not to be contradicted. Sometimes this is hard to put up with; respect shouldn't be confused with humiliation and contempt. Many doctors in Switzerland have little knowledge or recognition of advanced practice nursing roles. And the really good management job offers will always prioritise Swiss-born personnel.

You can lose your job if you so much as oppose a superior, who may accuse you of lacking loyalty. The nurse:patient ratio is luxuriously low, making the working conditions more than favourable when compared to France, despite their low thirty-five-hour working week law.[4]

The Swiss work a forty-two-hour week. Nursing schools are few and far between, and places on the four-year bachelor program are fiercely competitive with tough entry requirements. This means that Geneva's hospitals and clinics are almost totally dependent on bringing in outside workers like myself. I asked a high-ranking Swiss politician the reason behind this choice; he explained that housing nursing students in Geneva was beyond any hospital budget. A mid-career general nurse working full-time in a public hospital makes the equivalent of 85,000 pounds per year. A chief hospital physician can make over 2 million.

There was also another aspect of Swiss healthcare to which I was exposed, and it was a controversial one to many. But it was, and still is, one of the practices in Switzerland that I personally found both humane and ground-breaking – it is called 'Exit'. Exit is a voluntary assisted dying service. Death isn't taboo in Switzerland, far from it. If someone is suffering and heading towards life's *finale*, they can freely choose to knock back an anaesthetic syrup and fall into a deep, albeit lethal, sleep.

This evokes every ethical dilemma known to man, but I think it's a compassionate and gentle way to "go". It has often struck me that the way we allow vets to put down animals when

---

[4] This disastrous law fatally injured the French public hospital system. Jaques Chirac's government in the late '90s voted for an economic theory that considered hospital work time to be like a cake; let's make smaller slices so that everyone gets a piece! Nice idea, except that when more people share, the cake only gets bigger and more costly. To make matters worse, those who now worked less still went on strike or off sick just as often, being replaced by expensive agency staff. If we follow this economic logic to its extreme, the French should install a zero-hour week thereby creating an infinite amount of work.

they are suffering irreversibly is so much kinder than the way we allow some fellow humans to be treated at the end of their lives.

One thing I liked very much about nursing in Geneva was the undisputable requirement of being nice. It may sound crazy, but in some countries, you can be as rude and uncaring as you like without getting into much trouble at all. In Switzerland, however, the slightest complaint from a patient (or doctor) means you're out on your ear. The general attitude concerning Swiss healthcare was that kindness was essential. No smile? No job!

On the subject of jobs, I started my new one at the clinic amid a cracking crowd of guys and gals. I don't think I've ever laughed so much at work than with that lot. Many patients required sedation; general anaesthesia was reserved for retinal surgery, corneal transplants and people who were susceptible to leaping up off the operating table and racing outside at the first glimpse of a needle.

A general anaesthetic basically consists of checking your patient, putting in an IV and administrating oxygen, wiring them up to a monitor, pushing in the propofol etc., performing the intubation and hooking them up to a ventilator. After that, it's time to sit back, relax, keep an eye on the machines/patient and maybe chat with the surgeon about the case until it's time to wake them up for the extubation.

When it comes to sedating someone, however, it's a tad more complicated. The patient needs to receive *just* the right amount of medication (usually propofol mixed with morphine) to be relaxed and pain-free, to not move at all (even from snoring – we're talking microscopic surgery here), and to have a stable pulse and blood pressure – all this whilst continuing to breathe. Getting elderly folk to the end of their operation alive can thus be rather tricky, which is what the surgeons often had a little difficulty understanding. They simply didn't want their patients moving/talking/snoring. The problem is that nobody reacts the same way to the drugs; some fall fast asleep with a homeopathic dose, whilst others thrash around after receiving enough to kill an elephant.

Many of our ophthalmology patients had numerous comorbidities, making them fragile. Their heads are covered during surgery by a sterile drape hidden behind a big microscope, so we couldn't just ventilate them with a mask if they stopped breathing, such as during a knee operation, for example. I found myself needing to relearn old skills as well as new ones and having to perfectly master propofol: adapting dosages to each individual, then watching them like a hawk. It's a nerve-racking business; being rigorous was essential.

We also got very attached to our clientele, many of whom would come bravely back (most of us have two eyes) or for regular macular treatments, always good-humoured, gracious and grateful. We hardly ever heard anyone complaining, even when they had to wait for ages. Perhaps that's where the word "patient" comes from?

And the endless boxes of chocolates they bought us! If the entire team doesn't get diabetes later on in life, we'll be awfully lucky.

The patient turnover in ophthalmology is fast; we operated on around fifty or so patients per day. The pace alone required high levels of organisational and observational skills. I was never bored, and time flew. I was also under the false illusion that Swiss doctors would be a stern, humourless bunch. They're actually a great laugh, and Geneva was a real medical melting pot.

I've worked with all sorts: a talented if not slightly barmy Brazilian, a highly strung, high-maintenance Estonian, a sleepy, tree-hugging American who had been abducted into the Californian Moonie sect during the 1970s. I fear irreparable damage was caused. He was a "the earth is flat, aliens abducted me, and you really should drink your own urine" type. We were glad of his presence in an emergency, though; he literally bounced into action like a dozing dog that had just spotted a cat eating out of his bowl. There were a few grumpy gits as there are everywhere, but the vast majority of ophthalmologic surgeons, anaesthetists and nursing staff I met were great fun and extremely attentive to their patients.

And here, once again, the language quirks were a constant source of amusement to me. There was one that really tickled me after my first cataract case… and involved one of our many slightly deaf, English-speaking patients.

A plastic shield is put over the eye to protect it after surgery, especially for when the patient is in bed at night, rolling around and susceptible to post-operative injury. In French, this is known as a *coque rigide*.

"So, *monsieur*. You will now have to sleep with a RIGID COCK for the next FIVE nights, OK?" the surgeon informed him, loudly.

Not without Viagra, he won't, I chuckled to myself. He's ninety-five if he's a day.

Despite all of our efforts, occasionally, a patient *did* move during their operation. When this happened, the surgeon invariably shrieked, and all eyes in the room would turn towards the anaesthetic nurse in accusation. The first time this happened, I felt like Clint Eastward who had just walked into a bar full of Mexican assassins.

"Wi… will he be alright?" I asked, in traumatised terror, pushing more propofol into the IV.

"*Oui*. Yes." I was told. "But *you* get to choose the name."

"The name of what, exactly?" "The Labrador. His guide dog."

Just before I had a heart attack, they all started laughing. So *this* was Swiss humour…

Our surgeons spent their lives peering into a microscope.

Their obsession being that the patient looks into the light in order to centre the eye.

"*Voyez-vous la lumière,* do you see the light, *Madame/monsieur?*" This was repeated hundreds of times a day.

One day, Dr Montfort was preparing to carry out a cataract operation. Looking into the microscope, as usual, he asked the same old question, "Can you see a light, monsieur?"

"Yes, Doctor. I can."

Then, winking at me, he added, "I hope you can't see a tunnel too. That *would* be bad news!"

I stifled a laugh, which made me feel a little guilty, so I decided to reassure the patient during the surgery by stroking his hand. The simple power of the human touch is an amazing thing, as I said. His new lens was finally in place, and the scrub nurse was preparing his rigid cock w h e n he turned to me and said, "Thank you *so* much for holding my hand, mademoiselle."

Dr Montfort exploded into guffaws of laughter. "*Mademoiselle?* You think she looks young? *Zut alors.* Scrub the patient up again. The surgery has failed!"

Cheeky bugger.

In our profession, respect towards our peers and superiors goes without saying. But nurses should not feel obliged to bear intimidation. Not in *any* country. Maslow's pyramid applies to us all universally. Some people, however, will try any flattery to get in the doctors' good books (or bed).

I had a colleague, for example, for whom, if manipulative arse-licking were an Olympic sport, she would be the gold-medal world champion. Many times over. One of her more memorable brown-nosing episodes was when she told an Italian surgeon that she was in awe of him being able to work the microscope on both sides with both hands at the same time.

"How on earth did you become ambidextrous? It looks

terribly difficult," she cooed admiringly, accompanied by a fluttering of eyelashes.

"I had a professor at medical school," he informed us in his thick accent, "who told me that with both hands every morning and evening I should…" Stroking his bushy moustache, he searched for the term. Being Italian, his French was slightly limited, rather like mine. So, not finding the words, he decided to simply imitate the gesture.

Now… we all immediately understood very well that he was mimicking horizontally *brushing his teeth* with both hands, but, especially with the moustache, it looked so much like something from a gay porno film that the whole room went deathly quiet. Nobody was breathing. Except for the patient, luckily.

I believe that succeeding in not laughing and keeping a perfectly straight face at that point was one of the most difficult accomplishments of my life. And I wasn't the only one. Even our Titanic-tongued colleague was turning scarlet, biting her lip and looking like she was about to pee herself.

It was like one of the Monty Python sketches from the *Life of Brian*. A lispy Caesar introduces his best pal, Bigus Dickus, to the crowd. The centurion next to him has to contain himself or risk getting sent to the Colosseum and certain death.

None of us got thrown to the lions that day. It was a momentous collective effort, though.

They may not have lisps, but the French/Swiss *all* make the same mistake with the British *H*. I don't know why they insist on putting it where it shouldn't be… and omitting it where it should be. Nowhere is this more apparent than in an ophthalmology theatre which treats, as I said before, numerous English-speaking patients.

"'ello Mister Hedward 'ayfield."

"It's Edward Hayfield, actually. Good morning, Doctor."
"Gud moaning. So, during ze hoperation, you just 'ave to hopen your heyes, look hup at ze light and not move your 'ead. Hokay?"

"Hokay, Doctor."

The strange thing was that all these docs trained at the Moorfield's Eye Hospital in London. Surely then, they knew their H's from their elbows? Maybe they just think it's cute. Because, in a weird way, it sort of is.

Dr Montfort was telling me that during his training time in England, he'd had a young female patient come in with an unusually runny, inflamed eye. He took a swab to see what interesting microbes might grow on his petri dish. A mixture of chlamydia and dead semen was the last thing he was expecting. The follow-up consultation was executed quickly and with red faces on both sides. She was lucky; she could have gone blind! During the ensuing discussion, we concluded that there are only one or two ways to get semen on your cornea. Personally, I would have suggested keeping swimming goggles in her bedside table drawer. Or a ski mask, depending on the sperm count.

Another time, a patient wearing dark glasses and holding a Labrador on a lead arrived at the clinic, demanding loudly to be seen immediately.

"What seems to be the matter, sir?" asked Julianna, our lovely Portuguese secretary.

"It's my dog. It's got chewing gum in its ear."

"I think I misheard you. You said your dog has *chewing gum* in its ear?"

"Yes. Call my doctor at once, she needs to remove it."

"Sir, this is an ophthalmology clinic. For *people*."

In order to maintain calm, the surgeon was called to come and take a look.

Smiling, she was of the opinion that monsieur needed to

consult a vet.

"But you're my ophthalmologist, aren't you?" he argued.

"I am, indeed."

"So my sight is your concern?"

"Of course."

"Well, I can't get across the road without giving my guide dog instructions, can I? And now he can't hear me. Because of the chewing gum. So I could get run over... and *die*! Which would be all *your* fault." He shook a bony finger in her direction.

The doctor stood completely still for an instant, started to say something, and then seemed to change her mind.

"Kate," she said with a sigh. "Go and find me some long tweezers, would you?"

Work was going very well for Christophe at last. This was the first time I'd seen him allowed autonomy to utilise his many creative professional talents. The kids were enjoying school, and we were both extremely proud (in the way only parents are) to watch them turning into kind, generous, funny, hardworking and slightly crazy (but in a good way) young people. We considered this as the ultimate accomplishment of our earthly existence.

But life has a way of throwing you back down in the mud just when everything's going hunky-dory. The phone call came at 2 a.m. It was my brother, Chris, in London. Mum was dead. As of yet, there was no obvious cause. She'd been found by a neighbour who'd called 999 after no one had seen her for a couple of days. A police investigation had started.

The shock hit me hard. Really hard. I'd always known this day would come and, wrongly, it seemed, imagined it would be something of a happy relief. The world would be better off without certain people, and she'd been trying to die for ages, after all. This woman had neglected, physically beaten, psychologically crushed and then abandoned me. She'd lived an egocentric existence, throwing away husbands, children and friends like snotty tissues whenever it had suited her.

But she had suffered terribly too. Her horrendous experiences at the hands of abusive parents as a child had burned anger and self-hatred into her soul. She was incapable of loving anyone because she hated *herself* the most. Irreversible damage had been done both physically and mentally by her parents, followed by decades of various medieval-type psychiatric treatments involving electricity and hallucinogenic drugs. This had all led to multiple suicide attempts, not to mention drinking alcohol mixed with painkillers and sleeping pills over the years. She managed to fool so many GPs with *that* one.

"No, no. I never touch a drop Doc, honest! Just you go ahead and write that prescription…" They always succumbed.

I got the 8 a.m. flight from Geneva to London Gatwick, where I met my brothers. Tom, who I hadn't seen for decades, had flown in from Bangkok. We all drove together in bleary-eyed silence to her apartment and possible crime scene. A very gentle police officer met us and explained the situation. The necessary fingerprint swabs and photographs had been taken, so we were free to empty the place and take any sentimental memorabilia.

I remembered Mum telling me she was a twin and that her sister had died at birth. I listened at the time but never really gave it much thought – so used to the fact that half of what she told us was utter nonsense – till that day. When we opened her cupboards, there were two of the same, of everything: Clothes. Teacups. Books. Umbrellas. Slippers. Reading glasses… everything had an identical double. It was the freakiest experience.

A wave of pure sadness flooded over me. How can a life end like this? All alone, apart from a long-lost "imaginary" twin sister. Mum had written one of her PhD theses on twins, as well as several twin psychology editions. She had books upon books on her shelves about the Nazi twin torturer Josef Mengele. We were witnessing the enormity of her obsession. Perhaps it was all true?

Roger went through her laptop and discovered that she had been writing a book entitled *Vinegar Baby*. Why vinegar? Well, apparently, it was the main ingredient in an abortion concoction applied to sponges, widely used in the 1940s but which hadn't worked in our grandmother's case, despite multiple attempts at getting rid of our mother in utero. And, if we are to believe what Mum wrote, Granny insisted on reminding her of that failure every day throughout her childhood.

Mum described in the first chapter how she started to kill small animals that she found in the surrounding woods as a child. "I realised very early on that I had no feelings of remorse or empathy." According to the book, Granny stood in the dock in front of a jury, accused of trying to kill Mum when she was about thirteen years of age, along with her brother and sisters.

"Nothing gets rid of my daughter," she said, looking them all squarely in the eyes. "Not vinegar. Not gas. Nothing. Everything she touches crumbles. That's what happens when you force yourself into a world where you're not wanted. I never wanted her, so it's not *my* fault. If she hadn't been there, none of this would have ever happened."

How soul-destroying and damaging it must have been for Mum, a little girl, scared and vulnerable, to be faced daily with this murderous monster and extraordinary, unfounded guilt.

And yet I'd felt the same fear, lying wide-eyed in my bed as a child in the dark, listening to the sound of shouting, accusations and crashing, audible even through the pillow pulled over my ears.

Would she calm down and have a drink?
Would she leave for the hundredth time?
Or worse, would she come into my room?

My terrified eyes strained in the dark, looking out for a shadow under the door frame.

Further on in the book, my brothers and I came across this:

"I looked at my daughter Kate in the cot at the maternity, but just couldn't bring myself to love her... I knew I never would. Because she is me." I turned away at this point to hide the tears streaming down my cheeks.

Abusive relationships spiral down through generations unless consciously stopped. Hers was a story full of pain, hate and fear. The abuse she'd endured as a child laid down the foundation for her life; she was doomed without ever receiving the proper help she needed.

For me, however, it was a case of what doesn't kill you makes you stronger. And I do feel strong.

If my children decide to have children of their own, I'm convinced they'll be the best parents in the world. We're only really capable of loving another person once we've learnt to love ourselves, which comes through insight, strength of character and good parenting if we're lucky.

Mum also talked a lot in the book about her involvement in the Catholic Church, not only her faith and religious convictions but also several episodes where she was convinced she'd had heated conversations with both Jesus and the Devil, sitting at the foot of her bed.

There was hardly a mention of us, her children, either in her book or in the speech she'd prepared for her funeral. This hit Chris the hardest – he'd spent years trying to help her, making himself available day and night to listen. He was the one who had taken care of her each time her neighbours, the ambulance service or A&E, had called.

We talked about it and knew that the vicious cycle had to be cut. Rather than dwell on the sadness, we deleted the book and decided to focus on the future. This could only be done one way. Forgiveness brings peace.

And, when dwelling on death, I find a bit of humour helps too.

Good old Monty Python's, *Always look on the bright side of life* often jangles around in my head when times get tough, and it puts things into perspective:

> *Life's a piece of shit*
> *When you look at it*
> *Life's a laugh and death's a joke, it's true*
> *You'll see it's all a show*
> *Keep 'em laughing as you go*
> *Just remember that the last laugh is on you.*

We found out from the autopsy that Mum had taken her own life. In the absence of suffering from a terminal or debilitating disease, how lost and hopeless must one feel in order to make the decision not to see tomorrow?

She missed out on being close to her children, along with all the love she could have received from the grandchildren she'd hardly known. She missed out on the affection and tenderness that she could have reaped from her marriages with three lovely, kind men.

Depression ate away at her until there was nothing left. We should all be on the lookout for symptoms, both in ourselves and the people around us, and be ready to help. Good mental health is just as important as good physical health. Nurses have a key role to play, and I, for one, am happy that a few of our idolised young British Royals are showing such an interest in bringing these issues forward. In doing so, it may diminish the stigma and judgement attached to mental unbalance, which can affect any one of us during our lives.

According to the Samaritans, suicide is on the increase in the UK. France doesn't fare much better: 2.5% of girls between the ages of fifteen and nineteen have tried to kill themselves at least once. In the USA, suicide is the tenth leading cause of death at the time of writing.

After Mum's funeral, my brothers and I sat pondering over

our pints in a pub garden once the cremation ceremony was over. An elderly lady from Mum's church spotted us and made her way over to give us her condolences.

"Ah, you must be Kate," she reasoned, taking my hand. "Your mum mentioned you were a *nurse?*"

"Yes," I replied, quite surprised that I had figured in any kind of conversation between my mother and a fellow human being.

"She told me she was a little disappointed that you didn't become a doctor, though, dear."

Even dead, the woman made me grind my teeth.

"Be reassured," the old lady continued, looking round at us all. "God bless her, your mother is knocking at those pearly gates as we speak, and Saint Peter will be letting her in."

"He's probably more likely hiding behind a cloudy sofa," I retorted with a snicker. "Waiting for her to go away."

The conversation with my brothers then turned to *Vinegar Baby;* we questioned why on earth anyone would be interested in reading a book about the life of someone as unknown as our mother.

"Everyone's got something to tell, a unique experience, some opinion to give," I argued.

"You've had quite an extraordinary life, Kate," said Chris. "Why don't you write about all the stuff that you've done?"

"I'd read it!" laughed Tom.

"Pulling potatoes out of peoples' bums *is* rather entertaining," Roger added.

And the seed was thus sown.

"Maybe I'll dedicate it to Mum," I reflected. "She'd have liked that."

Tom took a drag on his cigarette.

"She'll come and haunt you," he warned cautiously, blowing out smoke. "The thing is, she won't even be scary. Just really bloody annoying."

I decided to risk it.

14. WHERE NOW?

Medication time... to meditation time

Whenever I talk to nurses, doctors and managers in the UK, the consensus is that the NHS needs help. One of my aims with this book was to use my experiences working within the healthcare systems of the countries in which I've had the opportunity and privilege to practice, taking the good and leaving the bad from each, in order to perhaps help come up with an ideal strategy.

These are my own, subjective opinions, and I know it's not smart to generalise. I encountered conflicting behaviour everywhere, and I am just one nurse out of so many, after all. But what the hell, here we go. Because for me, to not share these experiences would be a shocking waste.

Nursing shortage is a global problem. At the time of writing, in the UK there are around 40,000 vacant nursing posts in the NHS. This basically means that it is attempting to operate at 11% under the required staffing levels. So, over one in ten nurses are missing! Why? There *has* been a recent increase in applications, but the number leaving the profession is also, unfortunately, on the increase. To give an example, in 2014, 14,000 UK nurses graduated... but 8,000 retired and 18,000 left.

Nurses earn about 7,500 pounds less per annum on average than other graduate-level occupations. One nurse was quoted recently as saying "My children make more than I do. We have to resort to food banks and credit to survive." The main reasons given for leaving the profession in general are: income, stress, poor quality of care, workplace culture, bullying, work/life balance issues and being undervalued. The biggest age demographic of UK nurses is the 51-60 group; obviously heading for retirement and thus needing to be replaced. The key to solving the problem then, lies is retention. But how?

One of the things I have found hardest to accept in all my *own* days of nursing is that there are good health professionals, and there are bad ones. Some people wash their hands, some don't. Carers and curers can be kind or unkind. Surgeons can be calm and meticulous; others throw instruments around the room, like toddlers having a tantrum in their pushchairs. But in the end, no-one seems to be held accountable, whatever their behaviour. As students, we had to be nice to everybody in a senior position, bully or not, for fear of not getting our placements signed off. A nursing diploma can be like an ice lolly - you have to lick your way up to the top or risk it melting away.

As a patient, you might get looked after by a Florence Nightingale or a Dr House. Or perhaps it'll be a Harold Shipman or a Nurse Ratched… waiting for you with a sinister smile at medication time.

It's all too often a case of Russian roulette.

Hospital managers may be devoted to improving working conditions, patient safety and protocol. Or they may be narcissists, driven by cutting costs in order to make their personal annual bonus or simply hold on to their job. Sadly, the higher powers today are not always there to ensure care or deliver consequences but rather to reduce or even freeze budgets.

The days when the ward sister reigned over her obeying staff with a rod of iron (and none were more terrified of her than the consultants!) are sadly long gone. The wards were ship-shape, patients extremely well taken care of, and no one dared cut corners or be disrespectful. Widespread nosocomial infection and MRSA certainly didn't exist in the late '80s. I started nursing at the end of an era and have been a witness to the changing politics of health, since.

These days in NHS hospitals there is a serious quality issue;

there are high staff shortages as I mentioned, and working conditions can be so poor that people go off sick, burn out or leave. Conditions then degrade further… and we reach another stalemate. There is also little autonomy for junior staff nurses, now educated at universities, no longer obtaining a vocation-based, bursary-funded diploma but a degree following the infamous Project 2000 scheme. Nurses are graduating with a more prestigious piece of paper, perhaps, but without necessarily having focused or been evaluated on interaction skills, essential duties or vital common sense. They can feel lost, scared, sometimes disappointed.

Subsequent studies have found only very modest evidence of improvement in student nurses' views of how well-prepared they feel for their first placement. Many students don't finish their studies (about 30% in France). Of those who make it through, few remain in the profession for life. Little repayment then, for nine thousand pound-a-year fees. Despite these academic changes, salaries have been blocked for years. Many leave the profession disheartened and *nursed out*, often not long after qualifying. Staff nurses must pass regular, time-consuming tests in order to perform the most mundane, fundamental tasks. Skills that should have been mastered during basic training.

From personal experience, there are far too many queen bees and *definitely* not enough worker bees; often foreign nurses, buzzing around doing the hands-on, back-breaking work. 50% of nurses hired in the UK in 2022 were overseas graduates. Ironically, according to the Nuffield Trust, *non*-British/EU nationals are far less likely to leave the NHS, Britain's greatest treasure!

Carers can work extremely unsociable hours, including, of course, at night. One can earn a little more this way (some have no choice as a childcare solution), but the paltry remuneration increase doesn't make up for the fact that, according to studies, night duty may account for a 7-year decrease in life expectancy.

It's complicated enough for a lower-banded nurse to give someone so much as a headache pill without going through several layers of hierarchy – there are more grades in British nursing than there are in the army; it's one of those top-heavy upside-down triangle systems. By the time you get to the patient with their aspirin tablet, the pain's long gone. Or they've had a stroke, and it's too late.

Hospitals are managed like businesses; the most efficient, meaning the maximum productivity with minimum expense, get a governmental pat on the back. But since when is care measured by efficiency?

Bed/ward closures have to be the worst of their ideas. As soon as one is empty, some administrator closes it to "save costs." Predictively A+E gets backlogged, and patients get sent to wherever there's now space; the kid with a fracture gets stuck on the maternity ward; the elderly, confused lady gets dumped on the oncology unit... some poor souls spend the night in a corridor on a stretcher or even get transferred to a different hospital, miles away!

Staff are often told in this case to go home and use up their overtime hours, help out elsewhere or do evil "split shifts" (come in for the morning and evening, but go home between 11 am and 3 pm when it's quieter on the wards...). This lack of respect is one of the reasons nurses feel so let down. Why can't managers accept that during the rare decreases in activity, healthcare workers will at last have more time to take better care of their patients? A little breathing space is normal in any professional organisation. Cuts have to be made elsewhere.

Up until 2007, french hospitals were paid for by allocating an annual global allowance to each. This was judged unfair as certain institutions required larger or smaller envelopes than others. So along came the *Tarification à l'Acte,* or T2A.

Hospitals were now financed according to the number and nature of medical activities. One euro spent meant one euro reimbursed by social security.

It was deemed this would make managers more accountable. Patients were put into groups, and each group given a code...and price! (Depending on the diagnosis and treatment.) The idea was logical until hospitals started competing for patients requiring the highest reimbursed services. The race for productivity began, creating its own inflation and unfair distribution. Certain surgical acts were well paid compared to chronic diseases and psychiatric disorders. Obviously then, surgical units increased in number, whilst mental health ones were closed. Hospital directors could even barter for the cheapest implants, medicines and prostheses. So, no one was spared the consequences!

Ever since, healthcare costs have soared, but tariffs have remained stable. Doctors were thus forced to take on more and more patients, surgeons had to operate around the clock and then the 35-hour week just about broke the system.

A bunch of high-ranking medical and nursing professionals, led by an eminent French professor, famously contacted the health ministry to propose a more equal, logical system:

- Guarantee an <u>actual cost</u> reimbursement, taking inflation and population needs into account
- Give an annual dotation to each establishment in addition, according to their individual needs
- Senior healthcare professionals should be involved in all financial decision making
- Develop telemedicine consultations and ambulatory surgery where possible to reduce expenditure
- Always keep the staff: patient ratio to a number which permits absolute patient safety and comfort
- Regroup public and private activity in a pertinent way

- Nurses should only get redistributed to other departments with their full consent to avoid catastrophic consequences…

In June 2016, a young French nurse and mother-of-two sat down and wrote a suicide note to her husband. She had been moved off her usual medical ward to help out in the understaffed neonatal ICU; a place both alien and frightening to her. Wrongly convinced that she had committed a serious medical error on a new-born baby, she chose to end her life.

Unfortunately, I could probably fill another book with stories like this. Preventable suicides amongst healthcare providers sadly occur far too often.

Declarations have been made by UK politicians that the NHS will soon be up for sale to the US. That it will be privatised. That the conservative government and their "Trade Bill" prioritises profit over health.

In fact, patient data is a sought-after commodity by drug companies and is allegedly sold for about ten billion dollars a year. Where is *that* money going? The worry now, is that these same companies procure contracts to provide services to the NHS via their vast data resources.

So, could that be a good or bad thing?

Privatisation certainly generally helps save money by increasing efficiency. Add to this better functioning operations, the development of new systems and products, an increase in private capital investment, and you see obvious positive impacts. Cutting-edge medicine is often expensive and not available in the public sector.

Total privatisation, however, will *always* increase the gap between rich and poor, so should never be the goal of any cultured society. A public/private partnership, where taxpayers' money is used to help the most disadvantaged, could be envisaged instead, just like that French professor and his chums proposed. Fair prices for medication and prostheses need to be monitored and controlled. In many countries this happens at federal level: The USA, Canada, India and some parts of South America.

It's interesting to note that the WHO discovered that health programs which are supported at state rather than national government levels, are more effective in attaining goals.

The American system of private health insurance is clearly too expensive. Medicare and Medicaid, however, in theory at least, are two of its more positive aspects and could be exploited if the NHS *were* to privatise. Medicaid covers all people with low incomes, even for nursing home costs, whilst Medicare is standardised and protects all the over-65s, along with people with disabilities.

Another positive element that I witnessed in New York was the importance of the quality control director at each hospital; a position often held by a senior advanced nurse practitioner. Their role is to assess risks and develop strategies in order to avoid patient harm and improve clinical outcomes.

Two examples of this I've already discussed - actors pretending to be patients and the recruitment test for nurses – quality control is vital in ensuring integrity, safety and meeting all standards set by health authorities. It's also very much appreciated by nursing staff, often involved in the projects. Developments in care quality set boundaries, bring teams together and, in New York, made us feel like we were moving forward professionally.

Since when is nurse recruitment conducted by a computer server in society's supposedly most humane profession? NHS hospital HR makes up its mind whether to hire someone or not using an *algorithm* for guidance, probably invented by a non-medical geek and certainly without having initially met all potential candidates. I would never have gotten into the profession if they'd used this hiring method back then! The rigid IT system also possibly identifies the person they can get for the least demand on their budget, not necessarily the best suited.

I believe the NHS has lost confidence in nurses. Over the past thirty years, there have been undeniable advances in medicine and nursing; human beings living longer is one tribute to this. But the NHS and healthcare professions weren't always in the general disempowered and disenfranchised state they're in now.

I cannot pretend to be an expert, nor do I necessarily expect anyone else to agree with my opinions, but my experiences have given me a unique perspective which I wanted to share with my fellow nurses (and anyone else who may be interested!)

Covid-19 has thrown a light on the ability of different countries' healthcare systems to cope. Worldwide, an estimated 450,000 healthcare workers had been infected with the virus by June 2020, with over 600 nurses having died at the time of writing. Infection rates vary greatly between countries.

The American system failed miserably in the face of this pandemic. Eddy called me up, devastated. Dear friends and colleagues in New York were dropping like flies. As Barack Obama posted: "The breadth and magnitude of its errors are still too difficult to truly fathom, but America has failed to protect its people."

Despite considerable advantages in biomedicine, wealth, resources and scientific expertise, it was countries such as Slovakia, Thailand and Iceland that achieved downward curves, not mighty America. Chronic underfunding of and disparities in US public health are two obvious causes, along with government misinformation and ill-prepared hospitals. At the time of writing, according to the *New York Times* database, at least 68,000 US residents and workers have died from coronavirus at nursing homes and other long-term care facilities.

The dedication and bravery of nurses and doctors everywhere impressed and inspired the entire world.

"No one is refusing to work," said the Israeli government's Chief Nursing Officer, "despite the danger this puts them in. We even had 12,000 applicants from nurse students wishing to volunteer help on their days off."

The Organisation for Economic Co-operation and Development published statistics that ranked Belgium as having the worst mortality rates. The Belgians responded by saying that the reason was diligent counting by independent epidemiologists rather than mismanagement.

The Belgian government included all real *and* suspected deaths in their count, meaning patients in care homes who had died with similar symptoms but who were not tested. According to them, less than 60% of ICU beds were occupied at the peak. Why weren't the other 40% offered to its many neighbouring countries in difficulty, I wonder?

They did admit, however, to not providing enough protective gear for workers.

The French strategy to the "first wave" crisis was seen by many as draconian at the time. Schools were closed in March, along with bars, restaurants and even ski stations. Social distancing was advised as early as February. The nationwide quarantine that followed was extremely well respected; it was a surprise to all that the French could be disciplined. I think they even shocked themselves.

Access to information was simplified, and the health

minister made daily announcements and updates. Healthcare workers who weren't working or retired were invited to help. All non-essential surgical procedures were postponed. The private sector freed up beds and ventilators in solidarity. Some patients were transferred to Germany and Switzerland on specially converted TGVs. Yet France still suffered 30,000 deaths at this time amidst a mask availability fiasco and a lengthy economic lockdown, for which generations to come will have to foot the bill.

One of the most remarkable changes to French culture following the pandemic was the end of the cheek-to-cheek kiss or *bise*. Then again, this may not be such a bad thing. As a Brit, I was never particularly comfortable with such close, affectionate proximity to strangers. So it's not all doom and gloom after all.

And how did the Swiss fare?

Our chocolate-chomping Alpine friends were ranked by many as having the safest country to be in during Covid-19. The Swiss government relied heavily on personal responsibility and used scientific-based arguments rather than prohibition. I don't think that this strategy would necessarily have worked in England.

I remember seeing a headline from one of our classier newspapers in around 2015, showing a proud Englishman proclaiming he'd put nine Cadbury's cream eggs up his bum. By the way, I can confirm from nursing experience that this *is* indeed possible, the good news being they just trickle out when melted, so surgery isn't even necessary.

"How can we trust people like *him* to wear masks and social distance?" one British journalist asked, making reference to this particular article.

It's a fair point.

On the day of George Floyd's funeral, 10,000 people gathered in Geneva wearing masks and keeping a one-metre distance from the person next to them as a show of solidarity.

The sympathetic government turned a blind eye, despite the fact that this exceeded the three-hundred-person crowd limit. The event went by peacefully and without health-related consequences.

Unlike in France, Swiss residents were free to leave their homes without a permit system. Vulnerable people were simply recommended to stay inside. Switzerland lost 1,900 people to Covid, but hospitals were not completely overwhelmed and even accepted foreign patients. A Bluetooth proximity tracing app was on the cards in Geneva. The idea was to be able to trace people who tested positive and avert others with whom they had come into contact. As in France, the public and private health sectors linked arms in solidarity; however, the public sector took the private's olive branch with great reluctance. There is an infantile, silent competition between the two, each unwilling to admit they need the other.

We helped out as best we could in our little ophthalmology clinic. Unfortunately, this period also witnessed a rise in domestic violence during lockdown, perhaps due to frustration and the close confinement we were all subjected to. Problems and challenges in relationships became less avoidable. It meant that we had several cases of black eyes and subsequent retinal detachments to deal with.

At the time of writing, over 900 international healthcare workers have died of Covid-19 on the front line. According to the *Guardian* newspaper, there are likely many more non-documented cases. No worldwide systematic, standardised recording system exists. In any case, 900 names from sixty-four countries have been submitted to a memorial created by Medscape. Their ages range from twenty to ninety-nine. Of the named list, 40% were nurses and 30% died from lack of PPE (Personal Protective Equipment).

The International Council of Nurses' chief executive was quoted as saying: "Nursing looks like the most dangerous job on the planet right now." A pertinent reflection.

As in France and elsewhere, the UK made fundamental flaws concerning the central government's procurement and distribution of vital equipment, such as masks. The real difference, though, was the British government's hesitancy in taking the situation seriously, mainly for fear of economic loss.

The UK, along with the US, were theoretically the best prepared. Britain had even simulated one (code-name Cygnus) in 2016: a hypothetical influenza pandemic, which revealed a potential shortage of PPE and ventilators. The fact that nobody acted on this information is scandalous. These abstract risks were put on hold while Britain planned its economy for a potential no-deal Brexit. During the first wave, some nurses reportedly had to cover themselves in bin bags and wear bandanas around their mouths for protection.

Time magazine wrote an article accusing the UK of ignoring the WHO's guidance on Track and Trace identification and isolation, which obviously wasn't ideal or responsible.

British trainee nurses were pushed to the frontlines in March 2020 but received no pay as of July. To add insult to injury, parking charges for NHS staff were called for reintroduction towards the end of the pandemic, further challenging the relationship between health workers and the government – the same nurses and doctors who saved the Prime Minister's life. He'd better pray he doesn't catch anything else nasty!

The NHS and its workers took a beating but were adulated in the evening at 8 p.m. by the clapping public. This touching "thank you" from the people meant well. But it didn't stop anyone from dying. Or pay overworked nurses' childcare bills.

Having spoken to many of my fellow colleagues, I do realise that some are very happy and content with our profession. It's possible to diversify into many different sectors today, with numerous options being open to nurses who wish to further their career in the community, GP surgeries or academia. But I'm far from alone in believing that change is needed. Moving from a vocation to a professional status, nursing has, it would seem, sacrificed certain vital clinical skills. As I've already said, to become a nurse in the UK today, you must not only achieve very good A-levels but also pay those hefty university fees. Who in their right mind is going to pay so much to get a relatively poorly paid job afterwards?

The probable answer is people who have a true *vocation*... so why not leave it as that? Add common sense, a hardworking ethic and kindness, and you've got what I'm looking for when I hire staff.

Getting a sister's post in the '90s was referred to as "stepping into a dead man's shoes" because it was such an unattainable goal for a staff nurse that she/he generally had to wait for the sister/charge nurse in question to die. Nowadays, UK nurses can be relatively quickly upgraded to management level without waiting for them to have the necessary leadership experience and knowledge.

The French recently concocted a cunning plan to deal with their rapidly emptying nursing schools: they got rid of the entrance criteria. Now *anyone* can apply to be a nursing student. I feel that this is going a little too much in the other direction. Serious thought, the ability to work and study hard, a caring approach to life and, most importantly, motivation are essential when making this career choice. My personal theory on the recent increase of UK nursing degree applicants, aside from the attraction to certain overseas candidates, is the "wannabee-covid-hero" effect. Faced with the daily reality, however, the risk is disappointment and a change of heart. Maybe I'm wrong- I hope so. Only the future will tell.

The Swiss made the calculation of having very few nurse

training facilities and hiring foreign staff. This works because it's a small, central state surrounded by nurse-plentiful countries, all willing to make the trip across the border every morning for a more generous salary.

Many hospital workers in numerous countries today are what we refer to as agency staff. These guys are a great help and as valuable as gold dust when someone goes off sick at the last minute, or there's an unfilled vacant position on the ward. However, they have to constantly integrate for short periods into a variety of services; trying to find out where everything's kept is an extremely tricky task in itself. Agency staff generally earn more per hour, meaning managers are reluctant to hire them because of the cost, and so the wards and services remain understaffed. It's a vicious circle. And without generously increasing fixed-post nurses' salaries, it'll just keep on turning.

Some nurses make this "agency" choice in order to be able to work on the days and hours which suit them, plus to get paid that little bit more. All the moving around, however, does sometimes keep them from becoming a real part of the team. They can neither be expected to invest themselves fully in, find fulfilment with, nor be dedicated to a workplace where they'll only possibly be spending a few days. There is also often unspoken rivalry between them and the fixed staff, caused by the inequality in pay.

Nursing is still a chiefly female-dominated profession, although this is steadily changing. With the demise of the nuclear family, parents need extended help to achieve a work-life balance. Healthcare professionals work around the clock; night duty, bank holidays and weekends are the norm. So how do workers cope with childcare?

This needs to be on-site, free or heavily subsidised at the very least, as Amel so brilliantly introduced into the hospital where I worked outside Paris. This resulted in a significant increase in applications for jobs there. Ignoring the issue just leads nurses, who may really *prefer* to work at the local hospital, into moving to the better-paid private sector, working from nine to five in GP surgeries, or signing up with an agency.

Many people working in A&E today feel scared and vulnerable to violence. It's often not a safe place to be on a Saturday night, that's for sure. Attacks on staff by patients intoxicated by drugs, alcohol or both are common occurrences in some towns. Fewer and fewer nurses choose the emergency room, once so popular, as their place of work. In New York, there was a highly appreciated security guard at the door 24 hours a day. More costs, yes… but more nurses being happy to work in the ER.

To recap, then: NHS doctors are often overworked and burnt out, nurses are choosing more and more to leave or work elsewhere, nursing students are at university rather than on the wards, and the too-numerous managers are in the office having (yet another) meeting aimed at cutting costs.

So who's looking after the patients? Exactly. And, more to the point, what can be done about it?

The Ministry of Health, NHS managers, nursing university departments, and the NMC (who are responsible for setting standards) are all constantly looking into ideas to make positive changes to the system, and are far more qualified than myself in doing so. Again, very humbly, I just wish to offer my ha'penny-worth, my sole objective being to try and help by sharing my reflections based on experiences elsewhere.

First of all, no nursing utopia really exists as far as I have seen. Everywhere has its strengths and failings. What is obvious to me, however, is that wherever nurses are deservedly well-paid, empowered and respected, it leads to higher quality care. Purely because sufficient numbers of them *want* to work, and so there is a better nurse-to-patient ratio. It goes without saying that nurses' salaries in the UK need to be increased. And I'm not talking about a few measly quid either. They should be at least doubled, which wouldn't even bring them up to an average Belgian nurse's wage. Recruiting staff and students would then become so much easier. Faced with good working conditions and financial motivation, the void that is, I fear, otherwise inevitable in the near future, would be filled.

If we want to have good health workers looking after us when we get old, forgetful and, in the immortal words of those Ab Fab girls, "are dribbling into our incontinence pads", it's time to act *now*. Costly? Yes. But the cost of an almost "nurseless" NHS will be much higher.

In certain hospitals and clinics where I've worked, there's an end-of-year bonus scheme for people who've taken little or no sick leave. This may sound slightly immoral, but it works brilliantly in diminishing absenteeism! Human nature is often naturally lazy… given the idea of a nice year-end cheque, you force yourself out of bed and scurry off to work, even if you're not feeling like it. (Serious illnesses requiring time off are not included, obviously.) This saves health services, not to mention social security, an awful lot of money.

A meaningful assessment needs to be conducted over the future of nurses' education. Getting back to hands-on training seems essential to me. The hours and hours spent in the library writing research papers could rather be put to use learning how to put IVs in properly. Then people like Peter would perhaps stand a better chance.

Using one's spare time to research, write articles (nursing is scientific and evidence-based) or even learn a new language should be encouraged in our profession, of course; one of the great things about nursing is that you can pretty much travel the world to work, even if it's only for a year or two.

Should prospective students know it, perhaps this career choice would seem attractive to the more adventurous? If only I'd been able to speak French, how less difficult and embarrassing it would all have been! It is predicted, for example, that by 2030 sunny California (one of the best paid places for nurses, with great working conditions) will need to recruit 44,000 nurses. Just saying!

Some French institutions have quite recently had the bright idea of paying nurses' study fees in return for two or three years of work in their teaching hospitals once they graduate. A win-win situation.

A number of nurses will want to go further into academia, which is both understandable and necessary. Nothing has ever stopped a nurse from doing what interests them. But mastering practical tasks, developing compassion, anticipation and communication skills, and using common sense and logic in decision-making – these are the most important nursing qualities and the key to becoming an accomplished professional.

A huge difference that I have witnessed in countries outside the UK has been the absence of different grading. French, American or Swiss wards can be staffed by nurses of identical levels of responsibility, with one manager who helps out if need be. In New York, the whole team rotated as the boss. Nurses who have been there longer or passed further exams may earn more, of course, but this is discussed individually and based on merit. There is an integration period for new staff and an annual evaluation for each team member. If you want a pay increase, you'd better have a convincing reason or two ready! It shouldn't just be based on a rigid scale. Cutting out all these middlemen and complicated grading saves administrative bureaucracy and, ultimately, money. Money that could help fund a universally improved wage for staff. Speaking of money, a number of health care professionals would like to know where their NMC contributions go. Each year, membership costs 120 pounds per person; that's 120 x 732,000 in 2021, totalling an astonishing almost 88 million pounds. Could that money not be used to somehow directly improve working conditions? And where does all the carpark money go, too? Nurses shouldn't have to pay for that, on the contrary, they should be reimbursed for travel costs.

If nurses are trusted to make decisions, rather than having to ask someone senior (who then has to ask someone else more senior), they will gain quickly in autonomy, confidence, knowledge, motivation… *and* save time! No one should be asked to do something they're not comfortable with, of course, which is why the sister/charge nurse needs to be physically present in the team, getting their hands dirty too. Not in meetings all day with the office door closed. If learning goes back to being mainly ward-based, three and a half years *is* enough to learn the essentials and prioritise basic care. I'd like to share an example.

When I was part of the agency staff in a Cambridgeshire hospital, I spent a while looking after post-operative patients who had undergone major cardiac surgery on the intensive care unit. I had a lot of experience under my belt with an expert eye but was on a low grade with zero autonomy. I'm not complaining… I'd willingly accepted the mission; having come over from France it was all they had to offer me at the time. I was simply happy to be back at work and looking after patients again.

I knew about cardiac patient care and that acute abdominal symptoms after heart bypass grafts can indicate serious complications. One day as I arrived for my shift, a lady in my care was writhing about in her bed. She was nauseous, febrile, hyperventilating, and her tummy was distended and hard to the touch.

"How long have you had this pain?" I asked her.

"It came on suddenly in the night," she whimpered. "They told me I'm just constipated with the morphine. Help me, please, nurse. It's excruciating!"

Mesenteric ischaemia occurs when the gut is starved of oxygen for a time. The gastrointestinal tract is particularly prone to damage from inflammation and lack of blood flow. It becomes a race against the clock to avoid bowel necrosis (tissue death).

It doesn't take a Nobel Prize winner to work out the importance of someone immediately examining this patient, yet I was absolutely horrified that no one would come and take a look at her. I was too low a grade to speak directly to a doctor or sister, and my N+1 (immediate superior) was busy. I didn't have time for the whole hierarchy ladder fiasco; that would have cost valuable hours. I urgently needed a surgeon to just place their hands on my patient. Simple as that.

I hooked up some IV paracetamol (this helps relieve pain and gets the fever down) before drawing up a blood gas. These samples measure oxygen and carbon-dioxide levels, amongst other things, and are super quick and easy to interpret.

It was bad. My patient needed more oxygen, so I popped a rebreathing mask on her. Her CO_2 (which makes the blood acidic) was high, which explained the fast respiratory rate: it's the body's way of correcting too much acid. I sat her up with pillows to make breathing easier.

Running from room to room, I searched in vain for a white coat. I barged into the staff room, explaining my concerns and was told to get out; there was a meeting. Who did I think I was? It would be dealt with later. The annoyed on-call anaesthetist told me that anything on the body below the lungs wasn't her concern and to stop bothering her. Nobody I beeped was available; they were all busy in theatre. I remember feeling frustratingly helpless and wanting to cry.

An angel suddenly appeared in the form of a young, surgical senior house officer visiting a colleague on the unit. He was surprised when I grabbed him, but followed me anyway, intrigued and probably a little scared by my panicked expression. He only had to touch the lady's tummy to immediately grasp the gravity of the situation. He ran off to warn and prepare theatre as I unplugged the patient's perfusion syringes, grabbed a bottle of transfer oxygen, chucked her notes on the bed and swiftly wheeled the bed out of ICU, crashing clumsily through the swinging doors as I tried to steer it alone. They removed half of her small intestine, which was a major operation but saved her from a life of bags, tubes and no longer being able to eat real food.

I didn't get asked back to work on that particular unit. Persona non grata, big time. I didn't really mind; the priority was the patient. Always. Analysing the situation long afterwards, it's clear to me that each nurse's potential isn't necessarily fully harvested. Why? What a waste! We all have different things to offer, individual qualities and experience, and we should be working together as a *team*. We're not a herd of sheep. Perhaps health service managers need to get to know their crews better.

NHS protocol seems to be structured in an almost robotic manner. It's as if everyone's wearing horse blinders, just ploughing along, following the rules, keeping their heads down and never questioning anything. At least, that was my experience.

As for the illusion that talking to a doctor is somehow a great honour for a low grade nurse? That's ridiculous. They go to the toilet like the rest of us! In many countries, there's equal respect between nurses and doctors on every level; we're all professionals with different tasks and roles, trying to take good care of our patients. Interdisciplinary teams complement and can teach each other: we're all on the same side, after all.

Nurses should positively challenge protocol and, more importantly, be part of a team approach in developing it. Old fashioned ideas, protocols and procedures evolve; they're not written in stone… evolution and change are fundamental aspects of the nursing process and we shouldn't be afraid of that. Ambition to improve is a wonderful thing! Everyone in *any* partnership should be involved in making things better, together.

And even if nurses or doctors have just arrived from a different country, listen to them. They may need help.

Or they may actually be able to help.

Remember the good old ABC? Apart from being a catchy Jackson 5 tune, it also stands for Airway, Breathing and Circulation.

For years you were taught that if you came across someone lying innate and unresponsive, you called for help. You fished around in their mouth to see if there was anything blocking the airway. Then you had to establish if they were breathing or not by lying down on the floor next to them, having a good look at their chest and seeing if you could feel breath on your sideways-turned cheek. If there wasn't any, you blew air into their lungs through the mouth, nose or both. Finally, after checking for an absent carotid pulse for ten seconds, you started chest compressions, which were stopped now and then to recheck the pulse.

Some bright spark questioned all of this one day. *Were we wasting precious time?*

If you realise that every second that passes without getting that essential blood to the brain and avoiding asystole, (the unshockable heart arrhythmia), gives your patient less and less chance of survival… wouldn't it be best to say that when an adult victim looks dead (unconscious with no normal breathing) just start massaging their heart and don't stop? This is, in essence, what one of the recent American and European guidelines on the subject of basic life support says.

NB: If you ever find yourself in the presence of a victim of cardio-respiratory arrest, call for help. Then, if you are not in any danger yourself, immediately start the cardiac massage. For an adult, place the heel of one hand at the centre of the chest at nipple level, then put the second hand on top of the first. 120 beats a minute is two compressions per second and roughly the rhythm of *Staying Alive* by the Bee Gees… they need to be about two inches (5cm) deep.

It's best to interrupt cardiac massage for as little time as possible unless the victim comes round, so if you get tired, hand over to someone else before stopping.

If I may, I'd like to add a word or two about recognising a stroke victim. There's an easy word to remember: FAST. F is for *face* which may be droopy, or lop-sided. A is for *arm*, one of which can be weaker than the other (ask the person to raise both arms to see). S is for *speech*, which generally becomes jumbled and incoherent. And T is for *time*; the symptoms often appear quickly and you need to get help as fast as possible. These people are best cared for in specialised centres, which may not necessarily be nearby.

Even if you're not too sure of yourself, trying to help is much, much better than doing nothing at all. Anyone interested can easily find simple guidelines on the internet, or why not sign up for local Red Cross classes?

In any case, that bright spark I mentioned earlier probably saved more future lives than we'll ever know simply by challenging old ideas.

One might argue that without empathy, sensitivity, energy and kindness, you're in the wrong job as a nurse. But one might also argue that working thirteen-hour night shifts for shit money and zero recognition whilst suffering from burnout also means you're in the wrong job. And could explain the lack of energy! It depends on how you look at it. But whichever way, who is going to think they're in the right job as it currently exists? Not many people, I fear.

Nurses sometimes work in utterly appalling conditions. Before even considering the lack of staff and non-stop exhausting shifts, let's talk about slimy secretions, obnoxious odours and suspicious sputum specimens.

Perhaps you'll come across buckets catching the drops from leaky hospital ceilings or burst drains. "Careful, slippery floor!" signs do nothing to slow you down; you already have too much to do in not enough time, such as hunting for a drip stand, urinal, cot side, pillow or electric cable, all of which, amongst many other things, there are never enough of.

You may be organising beds – the eternal juggle of trying to fit more and more people into a confined and limited space – or charging around getting patients to and from theatre, X-ray, the labs or up to their chemotherapy sessions.

We mustn't forget all the pre-operative workups and post-operative prescriptions. There are thirty sets of observations to take, medications to administer, IVs to flush, and bags to empty and measure the contents of. By the time you reach the last patient, it's time to start with the first one all over again. But you can't do that because people are waiting for their bed baths and dressings to be changed. Endless telephone calls need answering, beeps and buzzers responded to, and always with a kind voice or patient smile.

Then there are regular, often impromptu ward rounds; you follow, pen and paper in hand, bending your ear to hear, noting down the new treatments, investigations and decisions being quickly made as the doctors move busily on. If you need a pen, by the way, you'd better bring your own to work; pens are almost as rare as spare beds. You suddenly realise something.

"Um… Doctor Baily! Come back! You prescribed Augmentin for Mrs Kavanagh there. But she's allergic to penicillin."

"Oh, gosh… yes. Well, I'll come back and change it later." Then the information system crashes. All today's nursing notes are lost. Again.

Patients' charts need to be up to date, or N+1 will have your guts for garters. Sick, bed-ridden or elderly people may need help to eat and drink (that's at least three times a day), and let's not forget they also need to go to the loo. People who, for whatever reason, can't move around need turning every two hours to prevent pressure sores.

Then there's a cardiac arrest in room five. He didn't make it, and now you're forty-five minutes behind. You need to prepare the body for the family who are on their way, and the student nurse under your care is crying – it's her first death.

Talking to patients? Comforting students? Listening to relatives? No time for that. The hospital director is only interested in cost-effective high turnover, and efficiency. You're late for the next set of obs, and there's a ward round in ten minutes. A confused Mrs Jones has pulled out her IV line for the third time.

Mrs Jones has Alzheimer's. You changed the IV yesterday, and it took three male colleagues to hold her down while you did it. She has been admitted with congestive heart failure and needs the catheter to administer lifesaving diuretics and vasodilators. You were rewarded with deafening screams, obscenities being thrown in your general direction and a scratched arm.

You realise you haven't eaten anything or had a wee since 10 a.m. It's nearly 8 p.m. Actually, it's a good thing you've had nothing to drink! If you end up with a urinary infection, no worries, Dr Baily can prescribe you some antibiotics. You've been rushing around on your feet for the last twelve hours. You think to yourself, Yes! Nearly time to go home… have a bath, supper, glass of wine and collapse before doing it all again tomorrow. Then the night shift calls; there's a traffic jam. She'll be an hour late. Blast.

Now imagine that in a "normal" nine-to-five office job: you get to work bleary-eyed after four hours' sleep to find your computer's not operating and your chair's broken, so you'll need to stand up all day. Lunch and coffee breaks have been cancelled, and the toilets are out of order. Your colleague is off sick, which means that your already heavy workload has just doubled. Extra pay for that? You're joking! You already only make just over the minimum wage, despite having a top university degree. You won't make much more by the time you retire, so you'd better get used to it.

The air conditioning has failed. Crickey, what's that dreadful smell? That guy over there has a scary look about him; you become nervous. He shuffles towards you menacingly. You turn to walk away quickly and fall on your arse in a puddle of dirty water. Ouch! Go and find something else if you're not happy, everyone's replaceable, you're told. You'll need to write down all your tasks for the day so as not to forget; there are so many.

Didn't bring a pen? Well, you'll need to go out and buy one then.

This afternoon they move you over to the accounts department; someone's gone on maternity leave and needs replacing. You never learnt how to do accounting? Oh well, you'll just have to pick it up. Don't get the numbers wrong, though. Stay focused, or you could end up in jail…

It just wouldn't happen. But this is the daily reality for nurses. Not always, but far, far too often.

Change has to come from the top. A government that really – as opposed to rarely – cares about the NHS is essential. It could start by naming someone who has actually worked and rolled up their sleeves in a hospital, as health minister. I don't know if Oxford-educated Edward Argar has ever touched a patient, apart from maybe shaking their hand during a televised hospital visit.

In stark contrast, Olivier Veran, France's young health minister, was an eminent neurologist at Grenoble's university hospital before getting into politics. France's healthcare system isn't perfect, but at least its workers may feel that the person representing them has some real understanding of their problems and needs. He also recently got rid of the silly *numerus clausus*.

However, as I said, it's no paradise for nurses by any means. The bonus that was promised to French healthcare workers for doing overtime during the height of the Covid pandemic was only partially honoured. Agency nurses, some working well over fifty hours a week on intensive care units during the first wave, were told they weren't eligible.

"We're not giving extra money to people who only occasionally come and help," the government told them. They were invited to the Elysée in Paris for a cocktail instead. Great. Probably left-over bottles of cheap booze from some recent head of state visit.

In France, 2.8 million workers are agency staff. Of those, 7% work in the healthcare sector. The NHS spends around 8 billion pounds a year on them! 4.6 billion pounds alone were spent on agency nurses alone over the past five years in UK health trusts; a totally false economy, the BMA warns. We need to fill the positions with fixed staff, so let's invest the money in retention and attractivity, instead. These women and men put their lives on the line, along with many others during Covid, only to be let down in the end. Do you think they'll be back to help during future pandemics? We can only hope so.

For the twenty years I've been nursing in France, there have been endless calls from the profession, under pretty much every government, to reopen beds, stop closing hospitals and hire more staff. This has landed on deaf ears every time. The resulting treatment of nurses and patients in the wake of Covid is scandalous.

"I told you so" doesn't really help. Let's just hope we don't have to say it again.

According to the French governing body for nurses, *L'Ordre National des Infirmières*, 40% of nurses want to change their profession. Since 2022, 57% have been in some form of burnout. Doctors aren't faring any better. One-quarter of available medical jobs in French public hospitals haven't been filled. Disorganisation, unattractive salaries, over administration, too many patients, heavy workloads and lack of future projects are the main explanations given. As one anonymous paediatrician put it: "Since I quit my job at the hospital, I eat better, sleep well and have stopped yelling at my kids all the time."

As for the UK, one only has to read the brilliant, *This Is Going To Hurt* by former obstetrician Adam Kay to understand the situation.

Surgeons are worried, even furious. The staff taken away from the operating theatre in order to look after every hundred Covid-positive patients in ITU meant that 3,000 programmed cases were cancelled. The lady who found a lump in her breast that needed removing will have to wait. Will the cancer spread? We don't know for sure, but the stress certainly won't help.

The patient who has severe bilateral cataracts and can't see has been put back six months. Will he fall down the stairs in the meantime? His resulting hip replacement will be on hold too, if that's the case. Or maybe he'll have an accident crossing the road, injuring others? The young dad with angina who needs coronary stents placing… maybe he'll be OK. Or maybe he'll have a myocardial infarction and not live to see his baby grow up.

The list is endless… and all a result of bad budget management and short-term vision over so many years.

I got chatting to a bunch of people on a plane from Paris to

London a number of years ago. They were a boisterous French surgical team headed to the UK for the weekend in order to carry out eight hip replacements; four per day. "The waiting lists are preposterous in England," they told me. "So they called us to come and help. We're getting very well paid and are happy to do it in our spare time."

This seemed to me to be a brilliant idea but for some reason, these cross-channel trips seem to have fizzled out. Trying to uncover the mystery, it appears the insurance companies on both sides weren't at ease with whose fault any surgical complications might be. If that's true, what a shame! This sounded like such a good solution all round.

Nowadays, inversely, increasing numbers of Brits resort to (sometimes dangerous) surgical treatments abroad amid long NHS waiting lists.

Preventative medicine should be at the forefront of care. A good surgical thoracic team can remove the poorly part of someone's lung rather easily these days. But wouldn't it have been less traumatic, less painful (and cheaper) if we'd helped them stop smoking? Or even better, if they'd never started. Nurses need to be visiting schools and explaining ways of improving healthy living from an early age.

I've seen fantastic cooperation between public and private services in several countries. In an ideal world, yes, we shouldn't need private clinics and hospitals. But in reality, we do. They take the load off overworked, understaffed public health centres and give patients a choice. It needs to become a strong partnership rather than a rivalry. They have much to teach us; surgeries tend to be much slower in public operating rooms, and it's not just because of the teaching context – observing a junior house officer suture up an abdomen is like watching grass grow. Having fixed, functioning, dedicated and quick transport and cleaning teams are just as important as having good anaesthetists and surgeons in the running of a surgical service.

Extubating patients in the recovery room, as in most private hospitals, also saves a lot of time.

If you can fit more operations into a day, you cut waiting times, you save money, and you optimise hospital bed occupation with a higher patient turnover. Especially as so much is now done on an ambulatory basis. But, in order to maximise utilisation, public funding has to increase, and private healthcare subscription costs need to be at a level where everyone can afford to use it. Hospital financial controllers may want to get their eyes tested (I can recommend a good ophthalmologist) because they don't seem to have very good long-distance vision. The NHS needs long-term solutions; administrators should listen to what nurses and doctors have to say when making investment choices, restrictions and prioritising projects. Those professionals on the ground, they might actually know best!

Why does the NHs cost more and more, then? An aging population, higher running costs, training new doctors and more expensive medicines are the main reasons. Paying nurses more is a small, yet vital, fraction. And an element which every government chooses to ignore, hoping it'll go away. They're just *nurses*, after all, they'll shut up after a while.

Whilst doing my master degree in Paris, we were invited to a presentation by the then junior health minister. At question time, being a big-mouth, I took the microphone and asked why French nurses are so underpaid, not expecting the following reply, especially from a woman:

"Because when the profession began, centuries ago, nurses were either religious women or whores. That image stays with us today and is compensated accordingly."

Please note that in Germany the average nurse's salary is 80,000 euros per year, in Denmark it's 87,000 and in Luxemburg 90,000. These countries are next door! But obviously don't view their nurses as prostitutes or nuns.

I'm surprised that nurse anaesthetist training doesn't exist in England. I'm sure that the reason must be cost, but there is a major return on investment if viewed from a wider perspective. You get someone autonomous to do (a lot of) the anaesthetic work but pay them less. Bingo! Immediately doctors are freed up from theatre to do their pre-operative assessments and post-operative visits, and to help out in A&E, the maternity ward and the pain clinic, to name but a few responsibilities.

Anaesthesiologists (doctors and nurses) wear many different hats and have many different functions. If there was someone readily available in hospitals to put IVs into patients who have difficult veins or are severely dehydrated, perhaps Peter and others like him might still be alive.

In certain countries, the general public is held responsible and accountable to some extent regarding their healthcare. I remember an American patient suffering from cirrhosis benefited from a liver transplant, but only after formally agreeing to cease drinking alcohol, with help. There would be no second chance. The same rules apply to lung transplants for heavy smokers.

In France, the social security debt just keeps growing, so they've had to make some changes since the Golden Years (*Les Trente Glorieuses*) – from the 1950s to the 1980s when nobody counted how much was being spent. Now, people pay upfront to see their doctors and are afterwards partially reimbursed. A trip to see your GP ends up costing you about a tenner, which is still extremely good value.

A French GP will see their patient generally within twenty-four hours of calling for an appointment. Pharmacies are open day and night in most towns. When you collect prescription medication, half a euro comes out of your own pocket. All "comfort" medication (i.e. not vital) is paid for by the patient.

Whatever their financial situation or health insurance policy (apart from the most disadvantaged), the patient contributes one euro for every medical consultation or biological analysis, two euros for hospital transportation and twenty euros per day for a hospital bed.

You can choose your GP in France (assuming they have a spare place), and you must go through them in order to get your money back or referrals thereafter. The idea is to stop people from going to see loads of different doctors. A personal card, *la Carte Vitale*, holds your medical details and is used for payments and reimbursements.

This takes the weight off the emergency room departments, as people know there's a good chance of getting a GP appointment quickly, but they'll be waiting for hours, even days, if they turn up at A&E with a sore thumb. Now there's a thought. Maybe people with sore thumbs should pay each time they go to A+E?

Around 10 million people in France are entitled to 100% reimbursement for their treatment. If they are on the predetermined list of the 30 or so chronic illnesses, such as stroke and diabetes, they may benefit not only from this but also be exempt from making up-front payments; it's the GP who contacts the state insurance in order to plead each case.

However, as I said, nowhere is perfect.

Somewhere around 2009 in Paris, I worked for a while in the operating room, critical care unit and ER of a large hospital when the director (Mr Wormwood Scrubs himself) asked if I'd also be the referral nurse for the blood bank. He was already getting a good deal as far as personnel go and decided to try and squeeze me a little more.

The blood bank is a room full of fridges housing various blood products in very strict conditions, ready to transfuse when needed. In general, hospitals permanently have platelets, fresh plasma and three or four bags of O rhesus negative blood for emergencies; the precious universal donor.

The other blood types are ordered and prepared on demand.

It soon became apparent to me that major dysfunctions were occurring at night. Hospitals are different places after the day shift goes home; the normally heaving, noisy corridors are creepily empty. Basically, no one was around after sunset who could really be judged to have competent transfusion skills. The anaesthetist knew how to, of course, but he/she was more often than not holed up in the operating room with the usual night-time accidental fractures and unidentified wedged anal objects. The nurses in ICU were trained but busy with their own poorly patients. The night manager finished his shift at midnight, so was of little help.

When dealing with a massive transfusion situation, it's always best to include two people, at least. One person carries out the final checks, and the other hangs the products up, often putting them through a rapid warming machine.

The problem, as I saw it, was not with theatres, ICU or even the wards. When you transfuse massively at night, it's likely to be on the maternity unit. Incredibly, French midwives are not all formally taught about blood transfusion. There are two lives at stake, for heaven's sake! Maybe even more… And despite my pleading, these *sages femmes* stubbornly refused to learn.

"We already have too much to do!" they said, which was probably true, let's be honest.

In obstetrics, mothers-to-be are often already relatively anaemic through dilution, as blood volume increases during pregnancy. This is compounded by a potential change in clotting factors and platelets (these make your blood sticky when you cut yourself; they form a clot so that the bleeding stops).

For various reasons, when women give birth, there's a risk that the uterus (a muscle) doesn't contract back down as it should after the baby and placenta have come out, leaving its large blood vessels wide open. Bleeding can be profuse, both internally and externally. The mother not only loses red blood cells, but her clotting factors and platelets are rapidly consumed, so clots no longer form. The bleeding thus worsens, complicated by the fact that quantifying the amount of loss is almost impossible. It is imperative to deal with the situation quickly and effectively.

We'd had a few near misses, but luckily no fatalities as yet. It was clear that we needed to hire an extra nurse at night and train them in blood product transfusion. The reply to my demand was a resounding, "*Non!*"

"The only thing. The. Only. Thing… that matters to me, Kate," Monsieur le Directeur said, looking straight at me with dark, soulless eyes, "is the budget. I haven't budgeted for this. And neither will I."

"Even if it means risking mothers' and babies' lives?" I replied.

"How many have died so far?"

"Well, none yet. But several nearly."

"I can live with that. End of discussion."

He turned his spindly spine on me and walked off.

Needless to say, my resignation was on his desk the next morning.

This story simply illustrates to me that the people in charge need to:

A   Listen to their teams.
B   Have some experience of looking after people.
C   Care.

This particularly awful manager did save money by not hiring a night nurse but lost one of his team members who was willing to take on four jobs. If we'd all put our heads together, I'm convinced that we could have come up with a satisfactory, practical solution.

The best manager I ever had? Easy. Sister Morag in Brighton, back in the '80s. Sister Morag's philosophy (imagine a strong Irish accent) was: "If kindness isn't in your DNA, you can fork off my forking ward!"

Whenever there was a minute to spare on her busy medical unit, she'd hide clues or try to trick us. If we won, we got an extra ten-minute coffee break.

"All nurses report to the nursing station! The four patients in room seventeen have gone down to X-ray. I've staged errors around their bed areas."

"Student nurse Kate!"

"Yes, Sister?" I jumped to attention.

"It's your turn. Get to it!"

There was a bottle of Coca-Cola and some chocolate Maltesers in the diabetic patient's locker. The security side rails had been removed from the epileptic patient's bed. Two full packets of paracetamol had been hidden in the coat pocket belonging to a patient with a history of chronic depression and suicide attempts. A large family pack of salted peanuts was on a hypertensive patient's bedside table. I raced back to the main desk with my arms full, feeling proud.

Sister Morag was a genius. She just wanted to help us to use our heads and become better professionals. She still inspires me after all these years. If nursing could be fun, rewarding and practical, as well as paid a decent wage, then our future generations would stand a chance to be cared for by happy, kind, competent people. It's as simple as that.

So, what happened to the Coca-Cola, paracetamol, Maltesers and peanuts, I hear you ask? They mysteriously disappeared… nowhere to be found. The perfect recipe for hangovers, though.

Believe me, I'm a nurse!

About the author

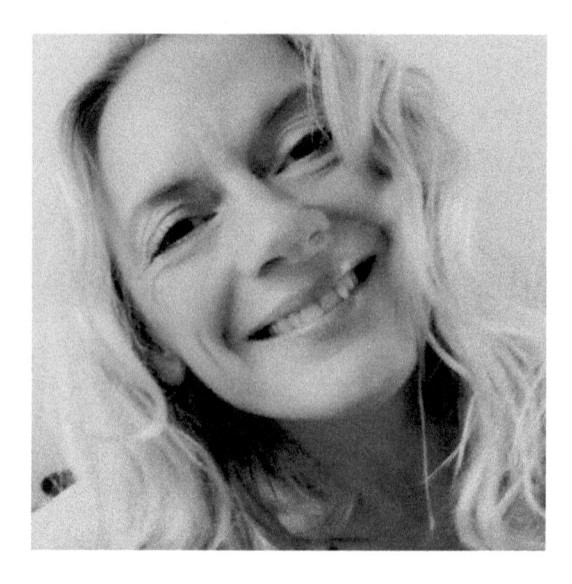

Raised in London's East End during the 1970s, Kate wrestled free from her mother's terrifying grip and went to Brighton Nursing School, where she discovered both the wonders and the struggles of being a nurse in the NHS. She has spent her adult years working in many different hospital departments around the world, and, against all odds, she's still at it. When not removing (mainly) inanimate objects from various orifices at the local hospital, she can be found scouring the internet for marmite and prawn cocktail crisps. Kate lives with her French husband, children and dog in Annecy, France. *You'll Never Believe Me, Nurse!* is her first book.